Evaluating Medicines

Medicines

PERSPECTIVES FROM A EUROPEAN REGULATORY AUTHORITY

EDITED BY

DS Slijkerman
JM van Ree
RTW Meijer
EMA Breeveld

C B **G**
M E B
College ter Beoordeling van Geneesmiddelen

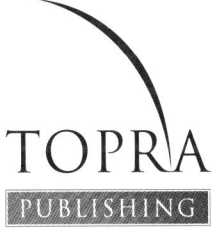

TOPRA
PUBLISHING

Evaluating Medicines
Perspectives from a European Regulatory Authority

Edited by
DS Slijkerman, JM van Ree, RTW Meijer and EMA Breeveld

Evaluating Medicines – Perspectives from a European Regulatory Authority is the English translation of the Dutch Agency of the Medicines Evaluation Board's book *Openheid van zaken – De werkzaamheden van het College ter Beoordeling van Geneesmiddelen*

Published by TOPRA Publishing
www.topra.org/publications

ISBN 978 0 9564943 0 6

Design and production by The Upper Room +44 (0)20 8406 1010

Preface

Galileo once said, 'Many are able to write in obscure technical jargon, but it is the ability of the few to write about complicated matters in plain language'. This could also be true for this first book from TOPRA Publishing.

The ability of the authors has been to explain, in simple terms, the intricate nature of European regulatory affairs in order for this complex process to be understood and appreciated. The efforts of the translators were not to alter the original esprit, but to offer an updated text which retained the clarity of the original. Written in the first place for the lay reader in 2008, this book has something to teach those who are starting a career in regulatory affairs, those who work outside of the European system and need to understand it more fully, and even experienced EU regulatory professionals who would like to have a view from inside one of our leading agencies.

Our sincere thanks are due to Dr Aginus Kalis, Executive Director of the MEB and member of the TOPRA Advisory Council for his enthusiastic support and for that of the whole Agency. The MEB has long expressed its commitment to transparency in the regulatory process and this book is proof positive of that commitment. The authors have expressed their views, which are their own and not necessarily those of the MEB or TOPRA, in a way that will greatly add to the appreciation we have for the work of a busy EU agency. Although written from the perspective of those who work in just one of the member states of the EU, the issues and challenges they discuss have relevance across the region.

I am particularly proud that TOPRA Publishing has achieved its first book, and even more so when this is a co-operation with a national Drug Agency like the Dutch MEB, thus assuring quality of content and practical 'hands-on' experience for us to draw from.

Launched in Stockholm in 2009 at the end of our Annual Symposium, TOPRA Publishing has its roots in the extensive and reputed educational experience of TOPRA. Over many years of training and educating regulatory professionals across Europe, and through the experience of producing the respected journal *Regulatory Rapporteur*, TOPRA has developed a sense of what our colleagues in this profession want and need to know. The launch of TOPRA Publishing and our plans for its future will help TOPRA deliver even more.

Our thanks go to the editors and authors of the chapters in this book for their dedication and openness. We are grateful to Carlos Langezaal (a member of our Board) and his wife Helene, who applied themselves to the translation, and to the staff of TOPRA Publishing who have brought this book to fruition.

Last but not least, thanks to you, our reader: I hope that this book will grow with you and that you can grow with this book!

Dr Paolo Biffignandi *TOPRA President 2009–2010*

Contents

1

The Dutch regulators

by Aginus Kalis and Ben Klijn

The Dutch Medicines Evaluation Board (MEB) was founded on 31 August 1963. It now comprises the MEB's executive branch and its board, which consists of a chair and up to 17 other members (doctors, pharmacists and scientists) appointed by the Minister of Health, Welfare and Sport. Board members are supported in their work by more than 200 employees at the MEB agency. The board secretary is also the agency director, and as such is the liaison point between the board and the agency, as well as being responsible for the quality of the agency's work.

The MEB is legally responsible for the evaluation, authorisation and monitoring of the use of human and veterinary medicinal products. It is authorised to decide on marketing authorisations (MAs) for these medicines in the Netherlands. The agency prepares these decisions as the executive board, and safeguards the consistency of the process. In the past, this role was mainly limited to national decisions (MAs solely for the Netherlands), but in recent years its dimension has become more and more European.

Functions of the MEB

The MEB's responsibilities and operating methods are laid down in the Dutch Medicines Act (Geneesmiddelenwet). Even before an application for an MA for a medicinal product is submitted, the MEB can be asked for scientific advice relating to all parts of the application dossier. The 'production process' starts when the agency receives the application for an MA. This application is evaluated and validated by a group of regulatory scientists. The result of such evaluations are generally presented to the board. Generally, because not every decision is original for a particular medicinal product, and in such cases references can be made to previous decisions.

Together with the MA, the content of the summary of product characteristics (SmPC) and the patient information leaflet (PIL) are evaluated. (A detailed description of the information that an SmPC and a PIL should contain is given in Chapter 2.)

After the MA has been granted, the medicinal product will be evaluated throughout its lifecycle on the market (this is known as pharmacovigilance, and is covered in more detail in Chapter 2 and Chapter 9). From this point in time, the emphasis is on collecting data with regard to side-effects, efficacy and misuse/abuse of the medicinal product for which the MA has been granted. One of the purposes of pharmacovigilance is the early detection of previously unknown or rare adverse events and interactions, as well as the identification of risk factors and the availability of information with regard to the prescription of medicines. If necessary, regulatory actions can be implemented.

The requirements for medicinal products are very strict. These firstly apply to the chemical-pharmaceutical aspects, where a product is tested to see that it conforms to all international regulations relating to pharmaceutical quality. The medicine is also tested for its effect in and on the human body, and possible toxicity. The latter still requires animal experiments. Finally, the medicinal product is tested on a broad group of patients for whom the product is intended. The decision as to whether the benefits of the medicinal product outweigh the risks is determined by the requested indication and the adverse effect profile. Certain adverse effects are more acceptable in, for example, medicinal products for cancer, as opposed to medicines for the common cold.

To make these decisions, the civil servants of the MEB need to be experts in the field of clinical evaluations, and also in areas such as epidemiology, statistics, pharmaceutical quality, etc. Another field of expertise at the MEB is regulatory affairs, where employees need to keep up to date with the continually changing environment of regulations and guidances. To be able to meet the demand for all these different expertises, the MEB has access to a great number of supporting offices.

The growing demand for MAs, and a growing emphasis on pharmacovigilance, has increased the need for staff at the agency, and consequently the number of people working at the MEB has more than doubled since 2002 (see Table 1). The addition of a Veterinary Medicinal Products Unit and a Novel Foods Unit has also contributed to the growth in agency staff numbers.

Year	Number of FTEs
2002	100
2003	112
2004	119
2005	146
2006	161
2007	184
2008	222

Table 1: Growth in the number of full time equivalents (FTEs) at the MEB, 2002–2008.

In 2008, the agency had around 275 employees (222 FTEs), working in five different offices located in various parts of the Netherlands. Experts are hired from the National Institute for Public Health and the Environment (RIVM), and there are collaborations with Dutch universities, academic hospitals, the Netherlands Pharmacovigilance Centre (Lareb) and other healthcare-oriented organisations. This wide-reaching structure enables an environment in which regulatory experts have first-hand knowledge of the most recent developments in their fields.

The MEB in Europe

MEB employees participate extensively in European organisations, working parties and exchange programmes. In doing so they increase their knowledge, and can share such knowledge directly and immediately with other stakeholders such as the European Medicines Agency (EMA), and indirectly with other EU member states. Because of this intensive cooperation and exchange of knowledge, the MEB ranks in the top five European offices that evaluate medicinal products.

The desire to achieve this ranking was first voiced in the MEB Strategic Business Plan 2005–2009. This of course is not the agency's only goal, as maintaining the high quality of the evaluation process and the safeguarding the interests of patients are primary. However, one consequence of being a key player is that the agency has influence on policy-making, and it enables the Netherlands to recruit internationally-renowned experts.

Future plans

In addition to the aforementioned aims and achievements, two further issues are being addressed by the MEB and deserve mentioning:

- Transparency: As society becomes more critical of the risks and benefits of medicinal products, governments and other stakeholders are demanding greater transparency from health authorities
- Converging technologies: In light of the convergence of emerging technologies with regard to pharmacotherapy, gene therapy, medical devices, novel food supplements and functional foods, new guidance and new regulations are required.

Transparency

The latest European legislation, 'Review 2001', highlighted a growing need for transparency in the decision-making process by health authorities. The increasing influence of the internet – enabling people to access information on medicinal products much more easily – required health authorities to provide up-to-date and accurate information to the general public.

This need was met reluctantly, as the pharmaceutical industry and some health authorities voiced concerns about making 'confidential' information more accessible.

However, the question arises as to whether much of this information is truly confidential. Individuals who regularly access financial and pharmaceutical news websites are usually better informed about companies' drug development pipelines than the average health authority.

In the interests of transparency, the MEB now publishes an abridged agenda and minutes of its board meetings on its website. It is expected that these documents will provide an increasing amount of information relevant to patients, physicians and pharmacists. The MEB's aim is to acknowledge and address the importance of transparency within the agency as an essential element of the organisation.

Converging technologies

The agency is an institution that invites the attainment of knowledge. This knowledge is distributed to a network of European registration authorities, as well as to national organisations. Paediatric medicines, orphan drugs and advanced therapies are three examples of where the MEB's dissemination of information on scientific activity can benefit society as a whole.

Current developments show the convergence of technologies such as medical devices, gene therapy, advanced therapeutic products, food supplements and functional foods. This creates a challenge for the MEB in its aim to cooperate more extensively with more organisations. Such activity also necessitates the recruitment of experts who are capable of following new developments and developing strategies accordingly.

In summary, the agency's activities have been proven to provide an essential contribution to the work of the MEB board. The board and the agency react swiftly and in unison to the changing needs of our society. In many areas they are indeed proactive, rather than simply reactive. As an example, in the field of quality management, the MEB is the world's only fully ISO-certified authority. It conducts a vast number of evaluations and actively participates in the European regulatory network.

2

How medicinal products get onto the market

by Pim van der Giesen

For centuries, pharmacists produced medicines and sold them to patients, sometimes with a doctor's prescription, sometimes without. During the twentieth century, the pharmaceutical industry increasingly took over the role of producing medicinal products and supplying them to pharmacists. Along with the products that pharmacists could make themselves, the industry provided them with new active substances, which were a welcome addition to the arsenal of existing medicinal products.

Diseases that were previously untreatable could now be treated or cured, thanks to the development of products such as antibiotics. Penicillin, for example, made it possible in the 1950s to cure patients with pneumonia within a few days, whereas before these patients often died.

Other infectious diseases spread by bacteria, such as sexually transmitted diseases (STDs) and wound infections, could now be treated effectively. For many years the pharmaceutical industry had free reign, developing and marketing medicinal products that were available to the public as long as they were sold through licensed pharmacists.

Halfway through the twentieth century, the notion grew that there should be more oversight of the burgeoning pharmaceutical industry by governments, to protect public welfare. Not every medicine healed the ailment for which it was recommended, and the saying 'if it doesn't do any good, then it doesn't do any harm, either,' did not always prove to be true.

There were many ineffective or even harmful products, and patients did not always get the best possible treatment. Regulating the situation, however, proved to be a long and cumbersome process. The need for regulation became obvious when the problems with thalidomide became known. Thalidomide, when used during pregnancy, caused severe birth defects, with limbs developed only partially or not at all. Thalidomide was originally recommended as a sleeping aid and to cure morning sickness, but resulted in thousands of children born with those severe malformations. The link between the malformations and the use of thalidomide was established in 1961, and development of the regulation of medicines was sped up, resulting in the creation of the MEB in 1963, as well as other drug agencies in Europe. A cornerstone of the regulations was the requirement for a marketing authorisation to be granted prior to placing a medicinal product on the market.

What does the MEB consider when deciding on a marketing authorisation?

When an application for an MA is submitted, the MEB checks if the product is of good quality, safe and effective. This seems logical, but it is not easy for a pharmaceutical company to prove that its product passes this test, and it is not always easy for the MEB to determine if the information supplied is sufficient proof. In cases of doubt, the MEB always errs on the side of caution, and refuses an approval.

The evaluation criteria consist of:

- Quality assessment: This involves assessing the pharmaceutical quality, which is proven by the specifics of the components, the description of the manufacturing process and the controls performed during the manufacturing process. The quality is also proven in the shelf-life specifications of the product as it is marketed, and storage requirements as specified by the producer. There needs to be a consistency in the quality of the medicinal product, and there must be no difference between different batches of the finished product.

- Safety and efficacy: These two criteria are inseparable. All medicinal products have desired therapeutic value as well as undesirable side-effects, although the latter may not occur in the same way or with similar severity in all patients. The acceptability of the side-effects and the degree of efficacy depend on the severity of the disease that the medicinal product intends to treat (the 'risk–benefit' balance). One example of this balancing act is with medicines to treat cancer, where more severe undesirable effects and a lesser rate of effect in the total patient population is more acceptable than for medicines treating mild pain, or for contraceptives. With the latter, only a very limited undesirable side-effect profile (in a limited population) would be acceptable, while efficacy should be ensured in almost the whole population.

Price is not a factor that comes into consideration for marketing approval, as this is not a scientific criterion. The risk–benefit assessment is primarily based on the safety and efficacy balance, not on the cost charged for the medicinal product.

What about PILs and other information on authorised medicinal products?

When the decision for an MA is positive, an SmPC will tell the manufacturer of the medicine under exactly what conditions the product can be marketed, and provides a summary with information on:
- Composition
- Therapeutic indications
- Dosage
- Contraindications
- Special warnings
- Use during pregnancy and lactation
- Effects on ability to drive and use machines
- Undesirable effects
- Overdose
- Pharmacological properties
- Pharmaceutical particulars.

The purpose of the SmPC can be summarised as follows:
- It serves as a 'contract' between the manufacturer and the registration authority
- It is the source for the PIL and the text of the label
- It provides information to physicians, pharmacists, and other healthcare professionals
- It serves as an accurate source of information when formulating advertising material.

The PIL is therefore based on the SmPC, and is intended as a source of information for the patient. As such, it needs to be written in layman's terms. Scientific information from the SmPC that is not relevant for the patient is not required to be included in the PIL.

The SmPC and the PIL can be found on the website of the national drug agencies (eg, www.cbg-meb.nl) and the EMA (www.ema.europe.eu).

The EU and medicinal products registration

The EU plays an important role in the regulation of submissions for MAs and, since 1995, in the MA procedure itself. The main goal of the EU is to abolish trade barriers. The first pharmaceutical Directive was issued in 1965, and stated that each medicinal product on the market in each of the EU member states should have a national MA. The criteria for this authorisation are the same criteria previously discussed, ie, quality, safety and efficacy.

This Directive was the first in a long line of regulations. The development saw the role of the national governments increasingly diminished. The reasons for this are twofold: first, pharmaceutical companies operate mainly internationally/globally; and second, knowledge is shared between regulatory authorities in different member states, including when issuing MAs.

In 1975, a second pharmaceutical Directive was issued, stating the information that needs to be provided when a company applies for an MA, and this was an important step in the harmonisation of the requirements.

The current process of marketing authorisations in the EU

In 1995, the European regulatory agency, the European Medicines Evaluation Agency (now the European Medicines Agency, the EMA), was founded. The purpose of this London-based institution is to supply administrative support to its six scientific committees and to coordinate duties that are held by national authorities, such as the supervision of clinical studies and the manufacture of medicinal products.

The six scientific committees are:
- The Committee for Human Medicinal Products (CHMP)
- The Committee for Veterinary Medicinal Products (CVMP)
- The Committee for Orphan Medicinal Products (COMP)
- The Herbal Medicinal Products Committee (HMPC)
- The Paediatrics Committee (PDCO)
- The Committee for Advanced Therapies (CAT).

This chapter focuses solely on the CHMP; the other committees are dealt with elsewhere in this publication.

The CHMP

The main responsibility of the CHMP is to formulate opinions regarding the issuance of, changes to, suspensions and withdrawals of MAs for medicines for human use. Only the aforementioned scientific criteria of quality, safety, and efficacy can be used. The CHMP opinions are sent to the European Commission for conversion into a binding decision.

Each EU member state has a member and an alternate member in the CHMP, who are nominated by the national governments for a renewable three-year term. It is the responsibility of these officials to coordinate the responsibilities and activities of the EMA and the national authorities. If it comes to an issue where voting is necessary, a simple majority of the members suffices. Alternate members vote if the member is not present.

There are also up to five co-opted members chosen among experts nominated by member states or the European Medicines Agency.

The CHMP has twelve permanent working groups to support. It also has groups to give therapeutic advice, known as scientific advisory groups (SAGs). All working parties consist of experts selected according to the particular expertise required.

The EU marketing authorisation

The EU MA is issued by the European Commission as advised by the CHMP. The authorisation is valid in all member states. The application for an EU MA is submitted to the EMA and follows the so-called 'centralised procedure' (CP). The CHMP provides a recommendation to the European Commission to grant or refuse the MA. This procedure is obligatory for biotechnology-derived products, for products used for rare diseases (so-called orphan products), and for products used for treating AIDS, cancer, neurodegenerative disorders and diabetes, as well as for auto-immune and viral diseases. This procedure may also be used for the authorisation of products with new active substances and for all other products bringing therapeutic or scientific progress and which are important for patients and animals at European Community level. This procedure may also be used for generic medicines applications once the data exclusivity periods granted to originator products authorised through this procedure expire.

If a medicinal product contains an active ingredient that does not fall into any of the aforementioned categories, the applicant may request to apply for the EU MA.

Obtaining an EU marketing authorisation via the centralised procedure

The EMA advises applicants to ask the EMA to check if their product qualifies for an EU MA before they submit their application. If the product passes this test, the EMA appoints a rapporteur and a co-rapporteur from among its members.

Rapporteurs are responsible for the assessment reports relating to the submitted data. To make their assessments, experts are available to them from the registration authorities of the member states. These assessment reports form the basis for decisions by the CHMP.

This committee is required to give its opinion on an application within 210 days of submission of the application. The 210-day period can be interrupted to enable applicants to answer questions posed by the committee. Applicants have the right to clarify any issues at face-to-face meetings, if they choose to do so.

The CHMP assessment report is based on the assessment reports of the rapporteurs, and is added to the CHMP opinion. The advice to grant an MA must also contain a draft of the SmPC, the PIL and the label, as well as a proposal for the product's delivery status.

To establish the delivery status, it must be determined if the product delivery is subject to medical prescription only, and also if there are restrictions to in-hospital use only, or that the product may only prescribed by certain physicians.

If the application is not granted, the applicant has the option to appeal the decision with the EMA.

If the recommendation is favourable, the SmPC, the PIL and the label all need to be available in every official language of the EU.

The recommendation by the CHMP is then converted into a decision by the European Commission to either grant an MA or to refuse the application.

The national marketing authorisation

National MAs are granted by the national authorities of member states. They are only valid in the member state(s) in which they were granted. They are used in cases where an EU MA cannot be obtained. To obtain a national MA, applicants usually follow the mutual recognition procedure (MRP) or the decentralised procedure (DCP), as described below.

Obtaining a national marketing authorisation through the MRP

The MRP is used when a company already holds an MA from one member state but seeks an MA in other member states for the same medicinal product.

The company asks the registration authority of the other state(s) to recognise its earlier MA, given by the first state, the so-called Reference Member State (RMS). The RMS is obliged to make available the evaluation report and all other related documents to the member state(s) concerned. (The MRP is documented in more detail in Chapter 7.) Another MA can only be denied for reasons related to public health, and the relevant member state must give its refusal within 90 days. If an issue cannot be resolved, it is forwarded to the Coordination Group (CMD(h)), details of which are covered later in this chapter.

Obtaining a national marketing authorisation through the DCP

The DCP can be used for medicinal products that do not yet have an MA in any member state and that are not required to follow the centralised procedure.

The company must submit the application in all member states that are concerned, and must indicate which member state has agreed to be the RMS. The RMS's responsibility is to compile a draft evaluation report on the dossier, and to distribute this with the drafts of the SmPC, the PIL and the label, to all concerned member states for their comments. Once the comments are integrated into the evaluation report it is sent to the applicant, who then has the chance to answer any questions that have arisen. If, at the end of the procedure, day 210, there is no consensus between the member states, the case is forwarded to the Coordination Group (CMD(h)).

The Coordination Group for mutual recognition and decentralised procedure for human medicinal products – CMD(h)

The CMD(h) comprises one member from each member state. It gets administrative support from the EMA, and meets monthly to discuss any problems that may have arisen while conducting the MRP and DCP procedures. The CMD(h) group must give a decision on an application referred to the group within 60 days. During this period, the applicant can clarify any issues in writing or in person, and if no solution can be found then the matter is referred to the EMA for arbitration by the CHMP.

How the CHMP arbitration procedure works

The CHMP considers the matter referred and issues an opinion within 60 days of the date of the referral. The CHMP assigns one (or more) of its members to act as rapporteur who is then responsible for compiling an evaluation report. The applicant can comment in person and in writing if necessary. If the CHMP decides to grant the MA, the opinion requires the same documents as in the case of a centralised procedure, ie, the SmPC, PIL and label. The opinion by the CHMP is then converted into a decision by the European Commission. Thereafter the member states have 30 days to grant an MA, if the decision is positive.

Reporting side-effects

Safety was the main reason for creating a licensing system to market medicinal products. However, at the time of a medicinal product's launch onto the market, knowledge about the safety profile of the product is limited. Typically only a few thousand patients have been exposed to the product during clinical trials in the development phase of the product. This means that hitherto unknown side-effects can come to light once the product is available to a broader population. Some of these side-effects can be severe. Since 1980 there have been many initiatives to protect public health by gathering information on newly discovered adverse reactions, or side-effects. One of these initiatives resulted in the founding of the Netherlands Pharmacovigilance Centre, Lareb (www.lareb.nl), which reports to the MEB and is also financed by the MEB.

The science and activities relating to the detection, assessment, understanding and prevention of adverse effects or any other drug-related problem is known as pharmacovigilance, and this topic is discussed more fully in Chapter 9.

3

Transparency – healthcare's new watchword

by Raymond Meijer

For decades, 'transparency' seemed to be a dirty word within the pharmaceutical industry. 'Confidentiality' was a useful synonym for secrecy – this, the industry thought, was how it was supposed to be, and the curious were kept at a distance.

That attitude has changed beyond recognition. Today, Europe requires all stakeholders in all its member countries – from drug developers to medicines evaluation boards – to expose themselves to public scrutiny at every turn.

The EU is demanding and stubborn: transparency and harmonisation have been added to the European dictionary. The MEB, and especially its past President, Frits Lekkerkerker, have been very conscious of these demands, and made great strides towards fulfilling them.

It is clearly important to inform healthcare professionals of all aspects in the evaluation of the safety and efficacy of a medicinal product. Which studies were used to obtain an MA? What precautions need to be taken when using this product? Which side-effects have been reported, and on which data are the contraindications based? For physicians, pharmacists and other medical professionals, key information (as detailed in the previous chapter) on any medicinal product can be found in its SmPC. However, while the summary is concise and unquestionably useful, it cannot offer full insight into the underlying data and documentation that were provided by the applicant when applying for the MA. Furthermore, not all studies conducted by a drug company for a particular product are published, and it is conceivable that negative data on any specific product may not see the light of day in the public domain.

This, then, is the situation in which we find ourselves today. There is a clear desire by all healthcare professionals for increased transparency in any scientific evaluation. Added to this, the MEB, as a scientific institution, is a strong advocate for transparency, as cross-evaluation by peers is highly valued in the scientific arena.

And it is not just the physicians and pharmacists who need additional information – patients demand to be informed too. Patients want to be involved in the treatment of their illnesses, and they also need to make their own choices with regard to healthcare beyond the doctor's office. In pharmacies and drugstores they can depend on expert advice, but in the grocery store they are left to make their own decisions. For these consumers, information needs to be provided in consumer-friendly terms.

Patients also benefit from objective information about medicines. Many sources, including the internet and the layman's press, are contaminated with incorrect or subjective information, which makes it difficult to distinguish myth from truth.

In the past, the risk of economic motives creeping into the evaluation process has often been highlighted, because of the increasing financial interests of the pharmaceutical industry. Critics who pointed at the influence of the commercial lobby on the MEB and its national counterparts could not be rebuffed, because the MEB could not provide the information to counter these accusations. Transparency will go a long way towards proving that the MEB does not consider commercial and economic factors when evaluating a medicinal product.

Before the implementation of Review 2001, the MEB was not mandated to allow anyone other than the MA applicant to access the reasoning on which the MEB based its decision. The law stated that the members of the MEB, as well as the board secretary, were sworn to secrecy. Evaluation reports were kept in the MEB safe. Review 2001 made significant progress towards transparency. Directive 2001/83, as amended, and Regulation 726/2004, as amended, require national regulatory authorities and the EMA to make evaluation reports publicly available. The main purpose of publication is to protect public welfare, but this goal needs to be achieved in such a way that the pharmaceutical industry, and the availability of medicines, are not hindered unnecessarily.

When an MA is granted for a new product, or changes to a marketed product are approved, a public evaluation report is published. In the latter case, examples of changes could be the widening of a product's therapeutic indications, or a change in dosage.

European legislature does not always require publication of a negative decision. Thus far, decisions to refuse an application have only been given to the applicant. European legislation[1] now states, however, that information on application refusals in centralised procedures, as well as the reasoning for these decisions, must be published. There are no guidelines about the format and the detail in which this information needs to be given. Directive 2001/83 does not give any directions on the publication of refusals of applications. [2] In April 2005, The EMACOLEX – a study group consisting of legal experts from the member states, members from the EMA and members of the European Commission – (see http://www.eu2007.pt/UE/vEN/Reunioes_Eventos/Outros/EMACOLEX.htm) concluded that the refusal of an application is a decision and as such needs to be published. The European Commission endorses this concept in its letter dated 25 May 2005, stating: 'The records should be made public after a final decision – authorisation or refusal – has been made. The records of meetings, including the votes and the topics of discussion could be made accessible at the same time as the public assessment report is published.'

The MEB has decided to publish its refused applications too, unless the decision is unrelated to public welfare, eg, in instances where the refusal is given for technical or legal reasons. On the other hand, refusals for MAs for new active compounds or for new therapeutic indications could be of interest to the public, and therefore more information about these products needs to be made available.

Evaluation reports need to be accessible to the public, although confidential industrial information must be omitted. Transparency must have its limitations. Data and documentation that have been provided by pharmaceutical companies to the MEB to obtain MAs cannot be published if they are commercially sensitive. Exactly what is considered commercially confidential information has been determined by the national authorities and the EMA, and not by the pharmaceutical companies. It is information with regard to the total quantitative composition and information regarding the preparation of the medicinal product. The quality of the medicine is safeguarded by the analysis that has been performed, and the evaluation board has the responsibility of evaluating the analysis and deciding on the product's safety. Pharmacological, toxicological and clinical data are not usually commercially sensitive and therefore can be published. Only details with regard to tests and analyses during clinical trials, as well as statistical computations, must be considered commercially confidential, unless they are already widely known. The MEB makes evaluation reports available that are stripped of this information, but it will also provide additional information on request, in order to clarify the information in the public evaluation report.

Until recently, the MEB has been restrictive in supplying information. It has only made an evaluation report available to the public if the MA for that product has been granted. However, the growing pressure of public opinion, as well as new legislation, has seen the MEB make the decision to publish public evaluation reports in cases of both refusals and approvals.

From all of this it is clear that there is a need to further identify what should be considered commercially confidential information, and that this needs to be done at an international level. Differing Freedom of Information Acts in the different member states therefore need to be harmonised. The EMA has taken the initiative on this, by compiling an overview of commercially confidential data that can play a role in European public evaluation reports, and of the regulations regarding access for the public to the documents being held by the EMA. [3] These principles are based on Regulation 1049/2001 of the European Parliament and Council, dated 30 May 2001.

The Heads of Medicines Agencies (HMA) are responsible for the harmonisation in the member states, to avoid conflicts with local regulations. Conflicts that do arise will ultimately be resolved by the European Court.

The pharmaceutical industry has protested at the increase in transparency being offered by the MEB. The industry raised many objections to the demands for information, both on public agendas and in meeting reports. As a result, the active compound, the pharmaceutical form, and the strength of a given medicinal product are all currently omitted from publicly available approval and refusal documentation. In light of this, the MEB is now working with the French authorities to take a first step towards harmonisation, because until full European harmonisation has been achieved, active compounds, pharmaceutical forms and dose strengths of discussed medicinal products will still be excluded from publicly available information.

Transparency, giving an insight into the reasoning of the decision-making process, will be increased in the future. However, this can only happen if the EU member states are willing to harmonise their Freedom of Information Acts, as needed, with the intervention of the European Court of Justice.

References

[1] *Article 12 section 3 Regulation 726/2004.*
[2] *Article 26 Directive 2001/83.*
[3] *Principles to be applied for the deletion of commercially confidential information for the disclosure of EMA documents Doc. Ref. EMEA/45422/2006, 16 February 2007.*

4

Who can sell which medicines?

by Diederick Slijkerman

In 2006, the MEB advised the Dutch Minister of Public Health on the criteria that can be used to distinguish between categories of medicinal products which are safe to be sold to the public without a prescription, ie, sold over the counter (OTC). The MEB initiated a project to define possible systems for classifying OTC medicinal products, and consulted several interested parties. The system the MEB eventually chose could also be used in other (European) countries. In Europe, each country can decide on its own system of OTC, since this system concerns national policy. However, all of these systems will have certain similarities, because they must be in accordance with European legislation relating to the boundary between prescription-only and OTC medicinal products. This chapter deals with the fundamental problems that the MEB had to confront when devising its system for OTC medicinal products and during the process of consulting interested parties.

Safety and the economy

The current system will determine which medicinal products can be considered for OTC qualification, and at which outlets they can be sold. Products that qualify for OTC status are those used to cure or alleviate minor illnesses that can be diagnosed without a professional medical consultation, like the common cold or headache, and they must be either topical or oral preparations.

For public health, it is important to maintain control when supplying medicines. The safety of medicinal products is highly valued by everyone, so much so that people tend to forget that no medication is entirely safe. Every medication has an active ingredient that can be harmful if used too often, or in the wrong way. Another risk is when an individual takes more than one medication, and unwanted interactions may occur. Finally, there is the risk that a particular medicinal product may have contraindications under certain circumstances, such as pregnancy. The starting point for a product to be considered for OTC qualification is that it is reasonably safe as long as the instructions in the PIL are followed.

The question of where patients should be able to obtain medicines has a long history in the Netherlands. For example, in 1853, surgeons were instructed to stop prescribing and handing out medications directly to patients. This was to be done only by pharmacists who, according to legislation in 1818, had sole responsibility for producing and delivering medicinal products. Pharmacists had a large financial stake in this, and whether or not it was for the benefit of the patient was not considered. This example illustrates that for centuries it has not just been safety and expertise which have dominated national healthcare. Financial and social factors have also generally been involved.

These social and financial factors are still important. The decision as to who will be allowed to sell medicines involves economic consequences, and hence politics and stakeholders can exert great influence.

This chapter discusses the dynamics of this process. It also explains how to determine which different categories of medicinal products can be sold, and by whom, which aspects and considerations may play a role, according to the MEB, in this process, and which ones may not.

The European context

In Europe, a two-tier system is used for the sale of medicinal products for human use. The first category is those medicinal products that can only be obtained by prescription from a physician. These medications are only available at pharmacies. The second category is medicinal products that can be sold without prescription, or OTC.

The criteria for prescription-only medications are determined by Article 71, Section 1 of European Directive 2001/83/EC, as amended. Medicinal products shall be subject to medical prescription if they:

- Are likely to present a danger either directly or indirectly, even when used correctly, if utilised without medical supervision, or

- Are frequently and to a very wide extent used incorrectly, and as a result are likely to present a direct or indirect danger to human health, or

- Contain substances or preparations thereof, the activity and/or adverse reactions of which require further investigation, or

- Are normally prescribed by a doctor to be administered parenterally (administration avoiding the digestive system, eg, subcutaneous, intramuscular, or intravenous).

Medicinal products must be prescribed according to these criteria if they contain new active ingredients. Supervision by a physician is necessary because there is a safety risk or a lack of clinical experience with these products.

The European Commission clarifies these criteria in its 'Guideline on changing the classification for the supply of a medicinal product for human use'.[1]

Within the European Community, OTC products are those that do not meet the criteria listed in Article 72.[2] They can be prescribed by a physician, but they can also be purchased directly by patients.

There are some European countries in which OTC medications are freely available, for example, the UK, Denmark, and Norway. These countries work with lists of compounds of medicinal products, but do not use general criteria according to which medicines are classified. The Netherlands has, in this respect, a unique system, in which medicinal products are divided into three categories:

- Pharmacy only (UA)
- Pharmacy and drugstore/grocery store only (UAD)
- Generally available, ie, can also be bought at supermarkets, gas stations, etc. (AV).

The Dutch Medicines Act lists the criteria for the first and third categories, and all medicinal products outside those two categories fall into the second category.

Criteria for an OTC system

The MEB's starting point for its thinking about medicinal products is that every medication carries with it the risk of side-effects, or adverse drug reactions (ADRs).

The MEB uses an adapted funnel model, in which the supply method (or legal status) is determined by the benefit–risk profile of a given medicinal product. The safety profile is not only determined by the active ingredient(s), but also by the pharmaceutical form and the way in which it is presented (dosage and package size) and the age group the product is intended for.

The safer the medication, the lower its place in the funnel. The model is adapted because the law states that the middle category should be a 'remnants' category. The first assessment is to determine if the medicine is too unsafe to be freely available to the public, so that it should only be sold in a pharmacy (UA), which will monitor the use of medicinal products by patients. The next assessment is to determine if the product is safe enough to be sold as generally available (AV). If neither of these categories applies, the product will qualify for the middle category, available OTC at pharmacies and drugstores (UAD).

For the category 'general availability' (AV), the law[3] states that this is only allowed if it is safe, considering the active compound, the dosage and the size of the packaging. The MEB has created additional criteria:

- The medication seeks to cure common illnesses that do not fall under the first category (ie, UA)
- The active ingredient has been in use for a relatively long period of time
- Use of the medication has a negligible risk of harm
- There is little risk of abuse or incorrect use
- The amount of medication per package is relatively small, and the package and PIL caution consumers on potentially harmful contraindications (eg, age group, lactation, pregnancy).

It is worth noting that the original proposed wording for the third criterion above was 'does not pose a disproportionate risk of harm', but Parliament rejected this proposal, as a consequence of lobbying by the association of drugstores/groceries. This association had an interest in keeping its own category, UAD (pharmacies and groceries only), as broad as possible. It took several actions against the other two categories, AV and UA, to protect its members interests and to influence corresponding decisions about classifications.

Examples of self-medication which is freely available in supermarkets and gas stations are paracetamol (limited to 20 tablets per container, and with a maximum of 500mg a piece), strepsils for coughs, aciclovir for cold sores (only as a cream) and alginates for stomach acidity.

The public exposure of policy decisions

In finalising their plans in 2006, the MEB held a public hearing for all stakeholders to comment on these plans. As a result of this consultation, the MEB added to its guidelines that the risk to patients must be minimised as much as possible by providing adequate information and guidance. However, the responsibility to read and follow the instructions lies with the patient.

In order to implement the plans at the same time as the new Medicines Act, the MEB compiled a concept list of compounds that would fall into the third category (AV).

The compromise of classifying most medications in the second category has meant that not much has changed, but when more medicinal products are made more generally available, the effect of the new Act will become more noticeable.

Nevertheless, MEB decisions on the classifications of medicinal products have already had great economic impact. As a result of its decisions, many complaints and objections were made. The association of drugstores/groceries has an interest in maintaining all products in the delivery status of pharmacy and grocery only (UAD), so they resented classification changes towards freely available (AV) and pharmacy only (UA). As mentioned earlier, the associations of pharmacies, supermarkets, gas stations, wholesalers etc, have economic interests that are affected by the classification decisions made the MEB. Indeed, all marketing authorisation holders in this sector have an interest in the classification decisions, as the pharmacy market is much smaller than those of supermarkets and gas stations. In the end, however, it is up to the MEB as a pharma-authority to defend the interests of public health.

References
[1] *'Notice to Applicants, A guideline on changing the classification for the supply of a medicinal product for human use'. January 2006.*
[2] *Article 72 Directive 2001/83/EC.*
[3] *Article 58 Section 2 Dutch Medicine Law.*

To register or not to register?

by Jan M van Ree

No medicinal product is risk-free – practically all medicines act as a poison when used in high doses (even water...). It is for this reason that not only must all medicinal products be evaluated for quality, safety and efficacy, and the risk–benefit balance be carefully weighed, but they must be used correctly: correct use and safe use go hand in hand.

Finding the balance

A medicinal product can only be authorised if it fulfils the three fundamental cornerstone requirements mentioned above. For the quality requirement, it is important that the manufacturing process is guaranteed, so that we can be sure that what is on the market meets the highest possible standards and that the product is always exactly the same, with no loss in quality. The product cannot contain any material that could be potentially harmful. There is increasing attention to the possibility of transmittable pathogenic germs, especially when human or animal material is being used. The use of animal material is subject to additional regulations. Some tissue cannot be used, and animal material must come from countries that do not have a history of TSE (transmittable spongiform encephalopathy).

The pharmacological-toxicological section of the dossier contains information on the effects of the medicine on animals. These preclinical studies are of great importance in determining the potential use of medicinal products in cases of specific therapeutic areas. They also offer insight on the pharmacodynamic profile of the medicine in such a manner that side-effects can often be predicted, as well as helping to determine the efficacy of a medicine in humans. One section of the dossier covers the findings of an extensive toxicological study, which can highlight potentially important side-effects of a product. In animals, research is conducted to evaluate the use of the product at single and multiple doses, at various dose levels (often much higher than in humans), as well evaluating any mutagenic, teratogenic or carcinogenic potential. All these data are considered when making a decision on the safety-efficacy balance. It must be mentioned that compounds screened by way of toxicological studies are often found at this point to have too many negative effects, so that further development is not recommended. And it is worth noting here that sometimes minor negative effects in animals can be major in humans, and vice versa.

The clinical section of the dossier includes information on how the medicinal product and the human body interact. Once a product is inside the human body, the body will try to rid itself of this (foreign) substance. It is important for effective and safe prescribing to establish the correct dosage by ascertaining how much of the medicinal product has entered the blood circulatory system. It is also important to know how the body metabolises the medication (again for dosage, but also for potential interactions with other medications and food).

The efficacy of a medicine requires extensive studies of its use in humans. These studies are usually randomised, double-blind and placebo-controlled. Double-blinding means that neither the researcher nor the patient knows if the patient is receiving the actual medication or a placebo. Even though the use of placebo in clinical research has been under scrutiny recently, it is still the gold standard to prove the efficacy of a new medicinal product. The possible therapeutic effects are determined by standardised and validated parameters. These late phase clinical trials only elucidate side-effects with a high occurrence, as the number of patients participating in clinical studies prior to registration is limited.

The decision

Deciding to allow an MA is never simple. How severe were the side-effects seen in human or animals? How important is the therapeutic effect, and in what proportion of patients was the product efficacious? Does it just treat the symptoms of the ailment, or does it treat the illness itself? The members of the MEB answer all these questions in the context of the disease and the use of the medicine. Different criteria are applied for a medicinal product used in the treatment of cancer than in a product used to treat anxiety or depression. Risk assessment and risk control are important considerations. Other, stricter criteria are considered for medicines in the treatment of pain that can be sold OTC. Important here are risk management and risk factors in the 'general use' environment.

The safety-efficacy balance of a new medicinal product is also compared with medicines that are already on the market. Information on this aspect can usually be obtained through comparative studies. If the efficacy of the new product is less than existing treatments, or if the risk of side-effects is greater, then a positive decision is less likely. The need for the medicinal product being evaluated is considered, but is not a determining factor.

The continuation

The MEB also determines the delivery status of the medicinal product. The options in the Netherlands were discussed in Chapter 4, and range from 'prescription-only' to 'generally available', where the medicine can be bought directly by the patient at many different types of outlet.

The responsibility for post-marketing surveillance, or pharmacovigilance, also lies with the MEB. This has also been discussed earlier, but to reiterate, the MEB avails itself of a variety of different sources to get this information: reporting by the public (patients and medical professionals); new clinical studies; and other data from various sources. Newly reported side-effects can be so severe that the MA has to be withdrawn or suspended. The MAH can also decide to withdraw the product from the market. In all such cases, the balance between safety and efficacy is the key consideration.

6

Oh happy days...

by Stan van Belkum

Thursday 8 March, 1990. While the Dutch worry about the soccer team who have just fired their coach, at the MEB it's just another day. In their office in Rijswijk, near The Hague, 40 employees process applications for new registrations, preparing for the monthly meeting. Evaluation of the new products is being done at the office, but also at hospitals all over the country. At the RIVM in Bilthoven, the data about toxicity are being evaluated. In Leiden, at RIGO (the National Institute for Medicine Research), quality checks are being performed, sometimes through laboratory research. There is close cooperation with the health inspectorate and with the European Pharmacopoeia in Strasbourg, France.

The telephone is the most important method of communication between Rijswijk and the other offices. The paperwork is delivered by courier, a few boxes at a time. Some employees complain that they cannot understand why so much documentation is necessary to prove that a medicinal product is safe.

The evaluation itself is a calm and precise process, resulting in a report that for different products can vary in length, but is 50 pages at most. These reports, and all sorts of letters, are being sent to the typing pool to be typed, corrected and typed again. The work at RIGO is revolutionary – they use Apple computers, and some people even have a personal computer. These computers use a disk that needs to be booted up each morning to start proceedings. In the typing pool there is panic; one day they will be unemployed because the computer will have taken over.

Management foresees that Europe will become a much bigger influence in the registration of medicinal products. The first steps towards mutual recognition have been taken. Policies are being developed, and people are considering opening up a European registrations office. The Dutch employees hope this office will be in Leiden.

In Rijswijk, they do not expect things to change any time soon. Europe tends to be even slower than the national authorities. They keep doing their work without much influence from the outside world. Patients and medical professionals are not involved in any way. Today, five medicines are being registered. There is a database called DATHUG (Databank of Human Medicines).

Thursday 8 November, 2007. What a difference 17 years makes! The MEB has moved to the centre of The Hague, near the Parliament buildings. By now it has around 250 employees. RIGO has disappeared, now incorporated into the RIVM. The working horizon has broadened: homeopathic, herbal, and veterinary products as well as new food supplements have been added. Nearly every application has a European aspect. The truly innovative medicinal products, for example those for AIDS, diabetes and products using biotechnological techniques, are directly registered for the entire EU through the centralised procedure. The location for centralised registration is at the EMA in London, UK. The idea of trusting each other's opinions more has been realised. As mentioned in Chapter 2, there are two new procedures, the MRP and the DCP, that make use of this principle. In the fields of paediatrics and rare diseases, there is a lot of European cooperation and many incentives.

Some previous safety issues have meant that the work of those who evaluate and those who register applications is receiving increased attention. There has been an increasing tendency to limit risk factors and ensure the safety of medicines. If a dangerous side-effect is reported, all sorts of bells and whistles will go off at many European study groups and working parties, and physicians, pharmacists and patients all over Europe are informed. The MEB plays an important role in Europe.

The dossiers submitted to The Hague have grown. For an application according to the centralised procedure, 100,000 pages (or their electronic equivalent) is not an exception. For generic applications, the dossiers are getting larger too. The number of applicable rules and regulations has increased significantly.

An important milestone was the harmonisation of the index as well as the content of the dossier in the ICH regions. (The ICH, or International Conference on Harmonisation of Technical Requirements for Registration of Pharmaceuticals for Human Use, is a unique project that brings together the regulatory authorities of Europe, Japan and the US and experts from the pharmaceutical industry in the three regions to discuss scientific and technical aspects of product registration.) Now, the pharmaceutical industry can use the same dossier – the so-called Common Technical Document (CTD) – to apply for a registration in the US and Canada, the EU and Japan. An electronic version of this document, known as the eCTD, has been developed to minimise the use of paper. Electronic systems have become increasingly important. Information and Communication Technology (ICT) and the internet have entered the pharmaceutical and regulatory workplace. The MEB has implemented its own website (http://www.cbg-meb.nl/CBG/en/). This web portal contains information about medicinal products, the latest safety information, and public evaluation reports, and is accessible to the general public. The PILs for patients and the product information for physicians and pharmacists are digitally available through the website. Email has become very important and, at the MEB meetings, everyone has a laptop with direct access to the central network in The Hague. Most piles of paperwork have gone. The number of meetings has doubled, since often an immediate response is required. It is expected that the workload and the number of people involved will increase further, as more information is made publicly available (see Chapter 3).

The future?

Thursday 17 September, 2020. It is busy at the office of LAGRA-9 (9th Local Affiliate of the Global Regulatory Authority [GRA]) in Utrecht, the Netherlands. At some point in time this was the building of the Dutch College, but they had their last meeting five years ago, before merging into the new worldwide system for registration of medicinal products, medical technology products, cosmetics and novel foods. There is pride that the Netherlands is an affiliate of the GRA. Now there are 15 'local' affiliates: seven in Europe, and those in the US, Brazil, China, Japan, India, Australia, as well as three rotating members from Africa.

Yesterday was the European video conference to prepare for today's worldwide meeting. All regional products have been discussed. Today, all of the new medicinal products and therapies will be discussed. All is set to go. The EU representatives of the Global Regulatory Board (GRB) are up-to-date and have reviewed all the available documents. The extensive computer analyses are being downloaded to the central system and compared with different regions. The comparison will be ready in an hour, and will then be discussed.

At the meeting, there are jokes about how, ten years ago, the efficacy of a new medicinal product was only studied in groups of patients, rather than in each individual patient. Individualised or personalised treatments, including dosage and composition of medicines, are common nowadays. Members praise themselves that Europe is central in this regulatory world. Their counterparts in North and South America and in Asia have to work either very early or very late. But it is still a tense moment when the Dutch representative enters her technically hermetically closed boardroom. She will spend the next three hours by herself, surrounded by every facility, all the information and online expert help. In recent years, there have been attempts to hack into the meeting, because of financial interests. This has led to maximum security but the meeting is still public, as it can be followed through various media. Pharmaceutical companies, patient interest groups, insurance companies and other financial institutions all listen in.

The meeting is being led from headquarters, the mainframe of the system. New products go first. The analyses are being explained, the most significant differences between the regions are highlighted, and ways to resolve these problems are suggested. Next is the session that can't be done by computer: the good old-fashioned discussions between the members about the material they have been shown. This is followed by a voting round, which will be analysed by the computer.

Next is the analysis of side-effects. Every abnormality in the trend analysis will be discussed, as well as individual cases that indicate special circumstances. All of this will need advice from the GRA.

Today, three new products and seven new therapies have been approved. Four decisions have been made about products that can no longer be used for specific genotypes. The meeting has been very successful.

7

En route to a European market for medicinal products

by Truus Janse-de Hoog

The mutual recognition procedure (MRP) (see Chapter 1) to register medicinal products in more than one EU member state was introduced as an optional procedure in 1995, before becoming mandatory three years later.

The MRP was based on the experiences of its predecessor, the multistate procedure. The intention of this procedure was for member states to follow the decision made by the first country to grant marketing authorisation. Member states, however, were allowed to decide differently or to alter the product information of a particular product. But this country-by-country freedom did not sit well with the EU's 'single market' principle, and so the MRP was born.

As mentioned in previous chapters, the principle of mutual recognition is based on the presumption that member states can adopt each other's decisions as their own, because the dossier requirements and the guidelines for evaluation are the same throughout the EU. The procedure is as follows:

● The applicant submits a dossier to apply for an MA in one of the EU member states

● After the MA has been granted, the applicant can ask the country concerned to become the RMS

● The applicant submits the same dossier with the same product information to the other member states in which he wants to obtain an MA. These countries are known as the concerned member states (CMS)

● The RMS sends the assessment report to the CMS(s) and, after confirmation that the application has been validated, the procedure can start.

The MRP takes 90 days. The only reason to refuse an application is if a CMS finds that there is a potentially serious public health risk. If this happens, the member states must do everything possible to come to an agreement about the dossier and the product information, with the help of the Coordination Group for MRP and Decentralised Procedures – Human (CMD(h)) or the Coordination Group for MRP and Decentralised Procedures – Veterinary CMD(v), if needed. The CMD(h) was set up in the revised Pharmaceutical Legislation (Directive 2004/27/EC amending Directive 2001/83/EC) for the examination of any question relating to marketing authorisation of a medicinal product in two or more member states in accordance with the MRP or the DCP. The CMD(h) also has the following specific responsibilities, as laid down in the revised Pharmaceutical Legislation:

● In case of disagreement between the member states involved in an MRP or DCP on the assessment report, the SmPC, the labelling or the package leaflet on the grounds of 'potential serious risk to public health', the points of disagreement are considered by the CMD(h). The CMD(h) uses its best endeavours to reach agreement on the action to be taken within the 60-day time period foreseen in the legislation

- To lay down, yearly, a list of medicinal products for which a harmonised SmPC should be drawn up, to promote harmonisation of MAs across the Community.

If the member states cannot come to an agreement, the application is referred to the CHMP for further discussion and possible arbitration. The decision from the CHMP is converted into a binding decision from the European Commission.

The development of the MRP and the role of the MEB

In the first year after its introduction, when it was still optional, the MRP had ten procedures, a number which grew significantly when the process became mandatory in 1998. In 2004 there was another considerable increase, as ten new countries joined the EU. Remarkably, this did not lead to significant problems, mainly because the new members were well prepared through training sessions and bilateral cooperation. The MEB built up a special relationship with the Slovakian agency. In 2005, 900 procedures for mutual recognition were initiated, and the MEB was RMS in more than 200 of these.

The MEB chose to be active as an RMS in Europe in 1995, by making a significant contribution to the scientific discussions. The agency decided to not perform its own evaluations of all sections of the dossier when it participated as CMS, but to refer to the evaluation of the RMS. In doing so, it applied the principle of mutual recognition fully while freeing up time to perform its own duties as RMS. In this process, the registration coordinators became very important, as they maintained contact with the other member states as well as with the applicant.

This European input has been promoted by the directors of the MEB. Dr C A Teijgeler, MEB director from 1967 until 1991 was very 'Europe-minded'. He previously worked for the CPMP (Committee for Proprietary Medicinal Products, the predecessor of the CHMP) and one of his mottos was: 'If it's good for the rest of Europe, why would it not be good for the Netherlands?' His successor, Mr Frits Lekkerkerker, was also very active in Europe. He soon became a member of the Dutch delegation within the CHMP, and became member of the CHMP in 2002.

The MEB's choice to be active as RMS and to be the first authority to evaluate dossiers has resulted in the agency's taking a leading role in the MRP. The European vision has certainly been important, as was the goal to promote the importance of a critical evaluation of the dossiers within Europe.

The role of the mutual recognition facilitation group

The CHMP, meeting at the EMA offices in London, UK, deals only with the centralised procedure and with medicinal products referred to the committee in arbitration procedures. Initially, there was no special group for the MRPs, but it soon became clear that there was a need for specially focused advice, and the MRFG was created. It held its first meeting in June 1995, also at the EMA offices. This group has played an important role in the execution of the MRP.

The description of the MRP in the European Directive was very brief. It proved necessary to provide more detail on how communication between member states should take place during the various phases of the procedure. It also came to light that many member states interpreted the requirements of a dossier differently. There was an obvious need to smooth the process of mutual recognition, and this task fell to the MRFG.

The MRFG does not have any legal basis. The chair of the group is from the country that is also the chair of the EU (a six-month rotation among all members of the EU, in alphabetical order). The MEB has chaired twice, in 1997 and 2004, on behalf of the Netherlands, and twice on behalf of Luxembourg, in 1997 and 2005.

Evaluating ten years of mutual recognition

The mutual recognition process was originally based on the presumption that member states were ready to accept each other's evaluations. If that were not possible, there would be a referral to the CHMP and, through an in-depth scientific discussion, a consensus would be reached. This would lead to a continued harmonisation of the European market. The outcome of the CHMP discussions would create a standard for the new dossiers. In reality, neither of the two presumptions came true.

Evaluation of the dossiers at a European level was only partly harmonised in 1995. Adoption of the approval by a different country was not automatic. It required more time and discussion at a European level to trust the quality of the assessment procedure in another member state. Another delay was the growing number of member states and EEA treaties. A third factor was that countries dealt differently in their determination of the necessary product information to be given to physicians and pharmacists, via the SmPC.

In particular, differences in the required SmPC information made it difficult to agree on a harmonised procedure. Many of the products using the MRP were generics, which created their own problems. When applying for an MA for a generic product, reference is made to the originator's dossier. However, the original dossiers were generally more than ten years old, and the SmPCs in the various member states were therefore very diverse.

The MEB also struggled if therapeutic indications were lacking in the generic product that were accepted in the original product. Because of the Netherlands' substitution policy, where pharmacists can substitute comparable medicines, the patient could miss important information. A European effort began, to harmonise the SmPCs of innovative products.

Referral to the CPMP did not happen as often as was assumed. In most instances when member states could not come to an agreement, the applicant simply withdrew the application in that country. This move was primarily commercial – the CPMP procedure took an average of nine months, and most companies deemed this too long. This meant that discussions to lead to more harmonisation did not occur often enough.

Industry complained that it was often claimed there was a potential serious public health issue, even when there were only minor differences between two member states.

Meanwhile, most member states made every effort to ensure the procedure was well run. Most of the European registration authorities deemed it important that this European registration procedure, as well as the centralised registration procedure, was successful, as the MRP leads to the issuance of national MAs. There was also concern that the EMA would conduct all of the registrations, thus decreasing the role of the national authorities.

The MRFG has played a key role in the continued development of the procedure. Even with continued objections on the grounds of 'potential serious public health risk', personal relationships between members were good, and they often came to agreement. Such agreements formed the 'Best Practice Guides'. The MRFG also issued guidances and Q&As for industry, published on their website.

However, it was obvious that there was still a need for changes in the law to really improve the procedure.

Changes after Review 2001 – creating the Coordination Group

In 2001, the European Commission began to evaluate the existing European procedures for the admission of medicinal products. This process, mentioned briefly in Chapter 1, was called 'Review 2001'. Industry and the member states were part of an extensive consultation process, offering information about their experiences with the European registration procedures.

One conclusion noted in the Review was that the procedure needed to be improved in order to achieve greater harmonisation in the market for medicinal products. In particular, the need was highlighted for scientific and procedural discussions between the member states regarding the applications.

As a result, a new provision was created, so that if member states did not agree on an application, the alleged 'potential serious public health risk' had to be brought to the attention of a new 'Coordination Group', even if the application was withdrawn in the country that made the objection. If the Coordination Group could not come to an agreement, the application must be referred to the CHMP for a binding decision.

The CMD was formed to replace the MRFG. This group has an official legal basis and a broad mandate to discuss all relevant issues, including scientific issues, concerning applications in more then one member state.

Within its remit, the decentralised procedure, covered in part in Chapter 2, was created, whereby a dossier is submitted simultaneously to the RMS and the CMS before an MA is granted. This makes it possible for all member states to discuss the application and come to the same decision.

The Coordination Group

The CMD, created in November 2005, has the following responsibilities:

- Disagreements between member states on whether a medicinal product poses a potential serious public health risk must be discussed by this group. All member states can participate in this discussion, but only the countries that received the application, the RMS and the CMS, can make the final decision. Countries must make every effort to come to an agreement. As all applications are national applications, there is no voting in the CMD, but the members are mandated by their national registration authorities to make binding agreements.

- The CMD decides on agreements about procedures and formulates guidances and Q&As for industry. As such, they continue the work of the MRFG.
- The CMD can publish an annual list of products to harmonise the SmPC.

In conclusion, the revised legislation, with the changes to the MRP and the new DCP, enables member states to come to agreement at a European level, with the help of the CMD if required.

As can be seen, the MRFG was very important in the development of the MRP and in reaching agreements among the member states. Weaknesses in the old MRP have been resolved by implementing the 60-day period by which member states must come to agreement or seek referral to the CHMP.

With regard to discrepancies in product information which can often lead to problems, the CMD publishes an annual list of products that qualify for harmonisation in the SmPC. At a European level, this means minimisation of the differences in product information for medicines with the same active ingredient. Changes to a product's information can be brought about by this process.

Most importantly for the success of the MRP, member states' national registration authorities actively support this procedure, giving their representatives within the CMD a mandate to reach mutually beneficial agreements.

By acting as the RMS, and by participating in scientific discussions, the MEB maintains an important role in Europe. As the RMS, the MEB ensures that the decisions taken are of high quality, and that public health is paramount.

The new MRP will lead to continued harmonisation within the European market for medicinal products. This is important because Europe has no borders, and there is much traffic between the countries. It is important that dossier evaluations are conducted by the national registration authorities. These authorities have the closest contact with their physicians, pharmacists and patients, and can most easily identify national trends and safety signals when products are on the market. Public health and safety needs to remain the starting point of discussions related to the granting of MAs. The CMD needs to ensure that the quality of medicinal products will be sufficiently safeguarded.

8

Centralised registration – Europe and the role of the national authorities

by Barbara van Zwieten-Boot

Medicinal products are considered goods in Europe. This means that there should be unrestricted shipping and trading within the borders of the EU. However, since such products deeply affect human wellbeing and carry great risks, they enjoy a special status.

In 1961, the first steps towards legislation for admitting medicinal products in Europe were taken. This resulted, in 1965, in the first Directive 65/65/EEC. This Directive made it mandatory for a medicinal product to be registered before it could be marketed. It took until 1975 to come to an agreement on how to realise this. In September 1976, the first meeting of the CPMP was held in Brussels. There were discussions at a European level about the admission of specific products. In 1987, it became mandatory to process applications for biotechnological products through the CPMP. However, the decisions were non-binding, and registration remained a national affair.

The CPMP created supporting discussion groups in 1976. The first such group discussed preclinical and clinical requirements. Later, in 1986, a discussion group was aimed at gathering biotechnological knowledge for Europe. Looking back, it can be said that those 20 years allowed member states to grow together and create a working system.

The centralised procedure

New legislation made it possible to register new medicinal products in all member states within one procedure, or to deny the application within the same procedure. The procedure was mandatory for some medicines, such as biotechnological products, while with other medicines the manufacturer had the choice of whether or not to use this new procedure. The goal of this new legislation was to make medicinal products equally available in all EU member states. The EMA was created (originally as the EMEA, the European Medicines Evaluation Agency) to achieve this goal. (The relationship between all the players is depicted in Figure 1.) As noted in earlier chapters, the agency's CHMP is responsible for preparing the EMA's opinions on all questions concerning medicinal products for human use.

Following marketing approval, subsequent monitoring of the safety of authorised products is conducted through the EU's network of national medicines agencies, in close cooperation with healthcare professionals and the pharmaceutical companies themselves. The CHMP plays an important role in this EU-wide pharmacovigilance activity by closely monitoring reports of potential safety concerns and, when necessary, making recommendations to the European Commission regarding changes to a product's MA or the product's suspension/withdrawal from the market.

With the extension of the EU, the make-up of the CHMP has changed, as detailed in Chapter 2. Today, members of the CHMP and their alternates must not only have a scientifically founded opinion, but must be able to liaise among Europe's individual

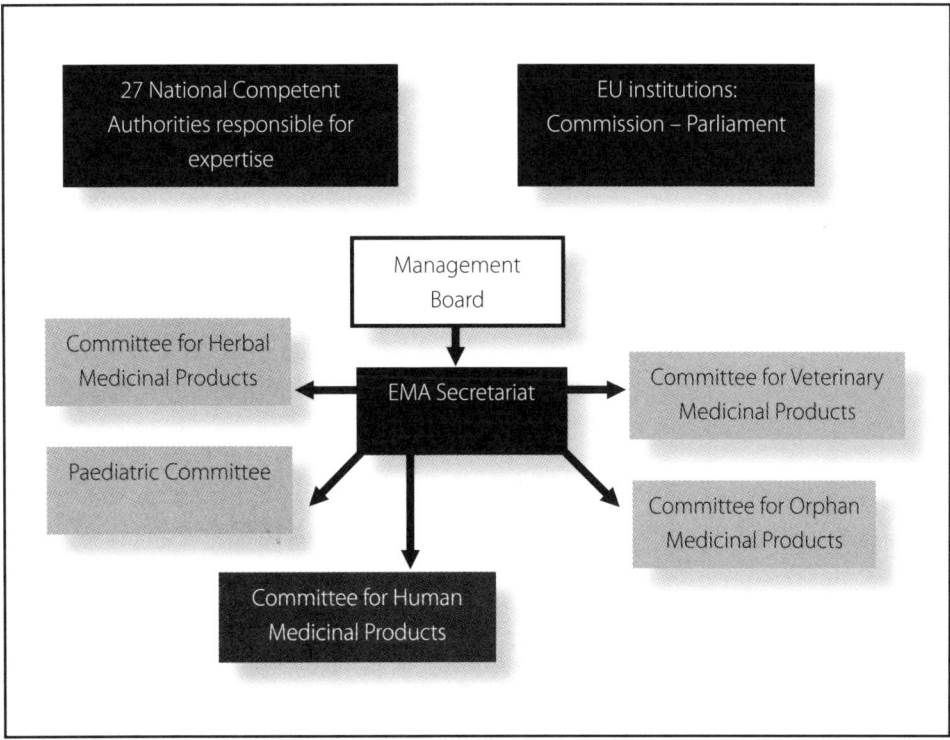

Figure 1: *The European Medicines Agency's key role in the current centralised procedure.*

countries. In the Netherlands, the MEB has a strong foundation in the community through contacts with universities and part-time physicians. Furthermore, MEB officials each hold jobs outside the registration process. The members of the CHMP bring a European perspective to the MEB and are able to contribute the Dutch perspective in their function as CHMP members. This system avoids the risk of an 'ivory tower' environment forming.

Evaluation teams

As noted in Chapter 2, each product discussed by the CHMP is assigned a rapporteur and co-rapporteur, chosen from attendees at the meetings. They each create their own evaluation team. Applicants will often choose to work with their own registration authority, but they can choose any European authority. As an example, the MEB has occasionally acted on behalf of Luxembourg.

Rapporteurs are chosen for their expertise and for the team they work with. This guarantees there is enough knowledge to handle the specific problems of a product. The Netherlands concentrates on the focus areas of the MEB, such as oncology, neurology, vascular diseases, neurologic and psychiatric diseases, but also on more general therapy areas such as vaccines and biosimilar products.

The composition of the team depends on the product and the procedure. In the Netherlands, a new product is assigned to a team comprising pharmaceutical, preclinical and clinical evaluators, among whom are those with pharmacokinetics expertise, methodologists, epidemiologists and people with experience in pharmacovigilance. If necessary, external experts are contracted. Teams are supervised by a regulatory coordinator, with the CHMP members having responsibility for the final decision.

Because the rapporteur's and the co-rapporteur's teams initially work independently, a unique system of quality control has been created. To avoid different explanations of the evaluation criteria, especially with the increasing EU membership, the CHMP has created a peer support system. EMA staff also assist in safeguarding the consistency of decisions.

Discussions about the acceptance of a medication will always remain. The balance between risk and quality, efficacy and safety, the key components for assessing every application, depends on the interpretation of the research. This interpretation will always be coloured by experiences with other products and in the field in general. Without the latter, it would be merely a paper discussion.

Working parties and additional expertise

The CHMP meets three to four days a month in London, UK. Much of the meeting is dedicated to discussions about products. Working parties have been created to make time to discuss management and recommendations for the development of new products and their evaluation criteria.

Some working parties have a general topic, such as the Quality, Safety and Efficacy Working Party. This group develops recommendations on the type of research necessary to reach an adequate evaluation of the risks and benefits of a product. These recommendations facilitate the development of products by the pharmaceutical industry, while harmonising opinions on the evaluations, and thus increasing the consistency of assessment reports.

Other working parties are more geared towards specific product categories (for example, biologics or vaccines) or toward product-orientated questions. To prepare for new developments in the fields of pharmacology and medicine, working parties have been created to study gene therapy, cell therapy and pharmacogenetics.

Members of the working parties are members of the national registration authorities. This gives the opportunity for knowledge-sharing, and builds relationships between employees from the different agencies. Figure 2 shows the network of working parties that has been created over time.

The CHMP can invite outside experts if required. These experts generally work in the clinical field, and give advice on questions related to a specific product. This is mostly in cases where the balance between safety and efficacy is not clear, and the CHMP is looking for a specific group of patients for whom the balance would be more positive. Another reason to hire an expert group is when a company appeals a negative decision.

To make the use of expert groups more transparent, and to be less dependent on ad hoc groups, six SAGs have been created for specific focal points, such as HIV and oncology. The members of these groups are nominated for three years. If necessary, additional experts or patient interest groups can be added to the SAGs.

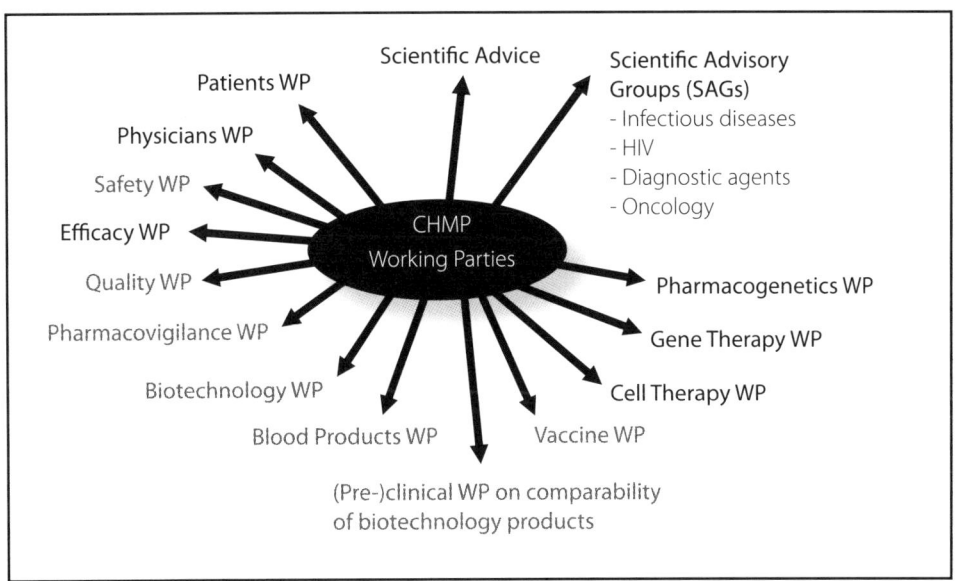

Figure 2: The CHMP's network of working parties (WPs) and scientific advisory groups (SAGs).

The role of the MEB

Before 1995, the MEB was responsible for submissions in the Netherlands – now it plays an important role in Europe. It is, and will remain, responsible for national submissions, with or without the MRP. The CHMP has responsibility for the registration and safeguarding of many new medicinal products; here the MEB has a more secondary function. One role is to ensure that the national and European evaluations do not have any discrepancies between them. The MEB also provides, like its European counterparts, the necessary factual expertise to keep the system going. It forms a link with Dutch society. Without this link, the evaluations would slowly drift away from daily practice.

Through the years, a unique system has been developed that does justice to specific medicinal products and to the desire that all the citizens of Europe have access to well-researched, effective and relatively safe medicines. It is up to the national authorities to maintain the expertise and to operate in a European context anchored in a national society.

9

Pharmacovigilance – stay alert!

by Kees van Grootheest, Sabine Straus and Chiel Hekster

While pharmacovigilance has been discussed briefly in earlier chapters, the aim here is to give a more complete picture of the many different facets related to the post-marketing surveillance of medicinal products.

The Netherlands has prioritised pharmacovigilance from an early date. In international literature in the first half of the 20th century, there was only sporadic mention of side-effects, but in 1951 Dr Leo Meyler laid the foundation for systematic attention to the side-effects of medicinal products, when he published a book on the side-effects of medicines. This book was translated into English in 1952 (Meyler's Side Effect of Drugs, Elsevier), and in 2006 the 15th international edition of this book – now considered a standard in the field – was published.

The birth of a great number of children with severe congenital defects caused by thalidomide in the 1960s opened the eyes of many to the fact that medications which were previously considered safe could have severe side-effects. The 'thalidomide affair' did not stand by itself, but it was one of many experiences with medicinal products that were popularly adopted but had unexpected severe side-effects.

Following this event, some European countries decided to create a registration system for medicinal products and a reporting system for side-effects. Thalidomide and other negative experiences with medicines also led to the formation of a system of post-marketing surveillance (PMS). This resulted in the new scientific field of pharmacovigilance, which is strongly stimulated by international cooperation.

In 1968, ten countries combined their experiences on behalf of the World Health Organisation (WHO). These countries were: the Netherlands, Sweden, Denmark, Germany, UK, Ireland, Canada, US, Australia, and New Zealand. In 1972, the WHO published a Technical Report with recommendations about the creation of a national reporting system, and reinforced the foundation for the exchange of reported incidents through the WHO Drug Monitoring Programme. A worldwide database was created to store information on side-effects. This database is still functioning, and is maintained by the Uppsala Monitoring Centre, a WHO collaborative centre.

Registration and monitoring of medicines – a necessity

The limited number and makeup of people who participate in any particular clinical trial for a new medicine are generally not representative of the whole population that will be using the medication. In clinical research, the aim is to measure the efficacy of the product for a specific illness. It is statistically and methodologically hard to measure an effect if there is a wide range of age, or other underlying illnesses, or concomitant medication use, for example, in the group of patients during the pivotal clinical trials. There are also ethical and practical objections to including children, women of child-bearing potential, pregnant women and elderly people in clinical trials. All this means that in many cases these population groups will not been included in clinical trials, so some side-effects will only become apparent after the medicinal product has been on the market for some time.

A system for pharmacovigilance after the product is registered has two components:

- Collecting and analysing the reports about possible side-effects of the medicinal product. Initially, it was primarily physicians who reported adverse effects, but later, pharmacists and nurses started reporting ADRs, and recently patients have also reported possible side-effects
- MAHs must report suspected side-effects of their product to the national registration authority – in the Netherlands, the MEB – or centrally, to EudraVigilance (a powerful database at the EMA).

There are three phases of follow-up if a side-effect is discovered: signal generation, signal strengthening and signal confirmation. A reporting system primarily discovers the side-effect (signal detection). This signal is strengthened by literature research or by previous reports in the Netherlands or internationally. This is where the WHO database plays a role.

Answers on the medicine-related relationship of a side-effect (signal confirmation) can only be given after testing the hypothesis analytically and experimentally. Key factors are the frequency of the side-effect, the risk factors, and the mechanism that forms the base for the side-effect. At the preliminary evaluations of a signal, all available data need to be considered and interpreted in their context. Most signals of unsafe medicinal products come from spontaneous reports. There is not always time and money available to conduct epidemiological or scientific research, and often it is impossible to do additional research because of time restraints.

The development of pharmacovigilance in the Netherlands

Because it is important to obtain knowledge about side-effects of medicinal products – knowledge which often only becomes available after the registration of a product and its availability to the population as a whole – reporting those side-effects is important. The Royal Dutch Medicine Organisation (KNMG) took the initiative by opening a central office to report side-effects in 1963. This office became known as the Bureau Bijwerkingen (Netherlands Centre for Monitoring Adverse Reactions to Drugs), which was later absorbed by the Lareb (Netherlands Pharmacovigilance Centre). Lareb is a governmental organisation for professionals involved in the gathering and analysis of data regarding side-effects of medicinal products.

Around 1990, the European Commission came up with a proposal for a revision of the Medicines Act. The notion of pharmacovigilance was introduced: a combination of a system of spontaneous reporting of side-effects and a monitoring/signal-detecting system by the pharmaceutical industry.

Inspired by this, the Netherlands Healthcare Inspectorate (IGZ) published a report on PMS in the Netherlands. It described all the research methods and came to the conclusion that there was a need for a national organisation to coordinate all PMS research. This resulted in the foundation of the aforementioned Lareb in 1991. In 1995, the Dutch Minister of Health,

Public Welfare and Sport (VWS) appointed Lareb as the national centre for the reporting of suspected side-effects of registered medicinal products by physicians and pharmacists.

A greater role for Europe

The European Directive on the granting of MAs for medicines, which came into force in 1995, saw many changes for member states. In terms of PMS, the EudraVigilance databank plays an important role as a data processing network and management system for reporting and evaluating suspected adverse reactions during the development and following the MA of medicinal products in the European Economic Area (EEA). The first operating version was launched in December 2001.

EudraVigilance supports in particular:
- Electronic exchange of suspected adverse reaction reports (referred to as Individual Case Safety Reports, or ICSRs) between the EMA, national competent authorities, MAHs and sponsors of clinical trials in the EEA
- Early detection of possible safety signals associated with medicinal products for human use
- Continuous monitoring and evaluation of potential safety issues in relation to reported adverse reactions
- The decision-making process, based on a broader knowledge of the adverse reaction profile of medicinal products especially in the frame of risk management.

The pharmacovigilance department of the MEB has many European dimensions, with special attention given to products for which the Netherlands has played an active role in the application process as rapporteur, co-rapporteur or RMS. All pharmaceutical companies with medicinal products registered in the Netherlands must submit periodic safety update reports (PSURs) which will be evaluated by the MEB. Safety information can be shared with the agency's European counterparts and, if necessary, with the US medicines regulatory body, the Food and Drug Administration (FDA).

A recent development is that a risk management plan (RMP) must now be submitted with any marketing application. In this document, the MAH must provide information on all known and possible future risks, and outline what plans are in place to deal with such risks. The evaluation of these RMPs is another task of the MEB.

Recent developments

The risks posed by medicinal products are gaining increasing attention. Expectations of the safety of medicines have risen, and the general feeling is that any risk is unacceptable. However, there are no medicinal products without risk. A side-effect highlighted and discussed in the media often appears to be an accusation, sometimes about the drug developer and almost always about the regulatory authority. This is more prevalent in the US, but also affects European society, triggering changes in pharmacovigilance procedures.

Patient reporting

Since 2003, patients have been able to report side-effects to the Lareb – the Netherlands was one of the first countries to introduce a patient-reporting procedure. Nowadays, reports by patients form a substantial number of all the reports received. The Lareb is researching the contribution that such reports make to the quality of pharmacovigilance. There is much international interest in the results of this research, because there is little experience with patient reports elsewhere. Patient organisations now have a seat on the Lareb, and within Europe these organisations are involved in the determination of policies. The EMA has also started consulting patient organisations.

Transparency

Transparency on every aspect of drug development has been discussed in some detail in Chapter 3 and elsewhere, but this aspect is particularly key in the pharmacovigilance arena. Industry, regulators and governments have previously been reluctant to share information on adverse events which come to light after a medicinal product has been launched onto the market, often believing that the publication of this kind of information might lead to unrest or panic, and would cause patients to stop taking their medications.

Under pressure from the European Parliament, however, clear regulations have been formulated that mandate the publication of safety data. Publication is important to increase public confidence in medicinal products and, where necessary, to restore it.

The Dutch reports on side-effects can be found at www.lareb.nl. The most up-to-date information on the adjustments of PILs and SmPCs as a result of these reports can be found on the MEB's website at www.cbg-meb.nl.

Intensive monitoring

In August 2006, the Lareb, with the MEB and the Royal Dutch Association for the Advancement of Pharmacy (KNMP), initiated a new form of pharmacovigilance: Lareb Intensive Monitoring (LIM). This is in addition to the existing system of voluntary reporting, and the experiences of users are essential to this initiative. For this system, pharmacists invite first-time users of a medicinal product to participate by completing brief email questionnaires. This enables the LIM to study methods of use and particulars of a product at an early stage. The LIM system is still in its infancy, but promises to take an important role in monitoring of the safety of a product.

What happens next?

Is all quiet on the pharmacovigilance front, now that we have all these European regulations? Probably not. The different aspects of pharmacovigilance as part of patient safety efforts will be at the centre of attention for some time to come. The public debate that followed high-profile withdrawals of particular drugs from the US market has shown that governments, and in particular the registration authorities, are viewed critically. The emphasis for the future, in both the US and the EU, is on creating greater distance between the pharmaceutical industry and registration authorities, as well as creating a division between registration and PMS activities.

Fortunately, in the past 40 years there has not been a disaster the size of the thalidomide affair. Timely detection of signals of possible side-effects, by analysis of reports and exchange of information, has played an important role in averting similar tragedies. Severe side-effects have been detected in time, and precautions taken expeditiously.

It is remarkable how much attention 'risk perception' has received, and how this can lead to unnecessary worries. This situation underlines the importance of continued efforts to do everything possible to minimise risks.

Bibliography

A C Grootheest, M N G van en Dukes, Leopold Meyler (1903-1973). 'Een pionier op het gebied van bijwerkingen van geneesmiddelen.' Ned Tijdschr Geneeskd 2003; 147(51):2526-9.

J A Lisman and J F F Lekkerkerker. 'Four decades of European medicines legislation. What have they brought us?', International Journal of Risk & Safety in Medicines 2005;17:73-9.

A C Grootheest, E P van, Puijenbroek. 'Pharmacovigilance in the Netherlands' in R D Mann and E B Andrews(eds) Pharmacovigilance, Chichester; Wiley 2007, 277-85.

J Langen, F P A M Hunsel, J L M Van Passier, L T W de Jong-van den Berg, A C Grootheest. 'Three years of experience with ADR Reporting by patients in the Netherlands', Drug Safety 2008 (in press).

J A Lisman. 'De toelating van geneesiddelen. Hoe effectief is ons system?', in Geneesmiddelen en Recht-Vereniging voor Gezondheidsrecht Preadvies 2006, Den Haag Sdu Uitgevers 2006.

The European perspective of pharmacovigilance

by Sabine Straus, Pim van der Giesen and Bert Leufkens

The side-effects of medicinal products have always caused unrest, and recent literature has seen many speculations about the cause of death of several great leaders. Alexander the Great could have died from side-effects of the herbaceous plant species, Hellebores, which is often poisonous, and it is said that Napoleon died of arrhythmia caused by quinine, a medicine the emperor had been taking. The death of some 'ordinary' people has played an important role in the attention to side-effects of medicinal products too. In 1848, a 15-year old girl died when she was anaesthetised with chloroform. Chloroform had been in use for a year, and it was preferred over ether as it caused less nausea. As a result of this death, possibly from ventricular fibrillation, *The Lancet,* a renowned British medical journal, created a committee inviting physicians to report deaths related to anaesthetics. These data were published in 1893; it could be considered a predecessor of the current spontaneous reporting system.

Rules and regulations

Progress in the field of medicine legislation and pharmacovigilance has mostly been determined by accidents or disasters. Adding diethylene glycol to a suspension with sulphanilamide (an antibacterial medicine) led to the death of more than 100 people, mostly children, in the US in 1937. It led to the Food, Drug and Cosmetics Act in 1938, an amendment of the 1906 Food and Drugs Act, tightening the regulations. Another key moment was the thalidomide affair in 1961, referred to in earlier chapters, when an Australian gynaecologist reported a 20% increase in birth defects, and the occurrence of the rare disease phocomelia (a malformation of foetal development where the upper appendage of an arm or leg is absent). It soon became clear that this was caused by thalidomide. This led not only to the foundation of the MEB in the Netherlands, but to the start-up in the UK of the Committee on Safety of Medicines, while in Europe it led to the adoption of the first directive on medicine evaluation.[1]

Looking at European legislation in this field, it is clear that there have been many changes and additions, as legislators have tried to adapt to new developments and the availability of new information. Rules were developed to streamline the tremendous amount of spontaneous reports of negative effects. Drug developers now need to submit PSURs, providing information on facts about medicinal products that have come to light after their registration. National governments have also had to deal with new regulations in the field of collecting, safekeeping and analysing spontaneous adverse event reports.

Legislature and Directives have been improved more than once. Despite these improvements, governments still have limited legal options to force MA holders to provide additional data to further support a favourable balance of risk against safety and efficacy. This is clearly illustrated by various publications showing that so-called 'postmarketing commitments' by companies are not always fulfilled.

A key moment in terms of modern pharmacovigilance came in 2005, when new European legislation introduced the concept of the RMP. This development illustrated the changing opinion of the registration process and the striving for a more proactive approach of pharmacovigilance. Registration of a medicinal product is no longer a yes/no decision, instead it has to follow a lifecycle approach. Both Registration authorities and industry must make an effort to estimate beforehand which safety problems could occur (on the basis of the available preclinical and clinical data), to monitor the product in daily practice after market launch and to reevaluate continuously the benefit–risk balance.

Another important instrument, as described earlier, is EudraVigilance, the database that contains reports on side-effects, which is as complete as possible. The intention is that this database will be a key source in identifying early and reliable signals of possible risks of medicines. There is also an initiative started to create a European network of cooperating pharmacoepidemiological research centres that can further study the reported findings. All these developments are leading to a European pharmacovigilance system that will keep evolving as society evolves.

The most important role of pharmacovigilance is the protection of public health by accurate and early detection of changes in relevance or severity of known side-effects. This knowledge is translated into actions that will safeguard continued access for patients who benefit from a medication, but also protect public health from avoidable or too severe risks.

Cerivastatin (Baycol) – a case study

On 8 August, 2001, Bayer voluntarily decided to remove Baycol, its cerivastatin product – an HMG-CoA reductase inhibitor used to lower the cholesterol level in blood – from the market in Europe and the US. Cerivastatin had been on the European market since 1997. The company withdrew the drug following reports of possible side-effects. It was reported that users of cerivastatin had an increased risk of developing rhabdomyolysis (a disease in which the muscle can deteriorate severely). An intensive assessment of the risk–benefit balance led to the conclusion that the medicine was effective in that it did lower cholesterol. However, it also came to light that there was an increased risk of developing rhabdomyolysis (the rapid destruction of skeletal muscle), a risk that further increased when the medication was used in higher dosages, sometimes with fatal outcomes. The evaluation also indicated that the number of cases of rhabdomyolysis, including fatal cases, during cerivastatin use is substantially higher than with other statins used at a comparable dosages. This situation was widely reported in the media, and 52 deaths were attributed to this medicine. Many patients who were on different medications for the same symptoms stopped taking their medications in panic. This led to many critical questions about the quality of the authorisation system and about pharmacovigilance. There were also many questions on the way the pharmaceutical industry reports adverse events to the authorities, and on how the authorities analyse and assess these reports and finally do or do not act.

There are differences between Europe and the US. In Europe, authorised medicinal products are reviewed every five years, something that is not done in the US. This review, however, did not result in the early detection of the side-effects of cerivastatin.

Another criticism was that the pharmaceutical industry, although mandated to report severe adverse events as quickly and completely as possible, struggles with this obligation. It is important for a company to carefully monitor its products, avoid unnecessary panic, and act effectively when something really needs to be done. However, this process happens in an environment which has great economic interests, liability claims and a justified emphasis on public welfare.

The cerivastatin case emphasises the importance of reporting side-effects by professionals in the field and by patients as primary sources of information on the balance between the risk and benefit of a medicinal product.

Rofecoxib – the Vioxx affair

In 2004, the world was shocked by the rofecoxib (Vioxx) affair, which may well be the third key moment in modern pharmacovigilance. In summary, rofecoxib was registered in 1999 for treating osteoarthritis pain, but when the affair came to light in 2004, it seemed that there was an increased risk of myocardial infarction (heart attacks). It was a medication in a new category of medications, known as the selective COX-2 inhibitors, with a similar effect on pain treatment as the older nonsteroidal anti-inflammatory drugs (NSAIDs) and was marketed as a safer alternative, as there was less damage to the intestines (gastrointestinal bleeding). In many publications, concern was voiced about the role the pharmaceutical industry plays in safeguarding the balance between risk and benefit. The accusation was that the drug developer, Merck, did not act quickly enough when it heard about the problems. Merck conducted an extensive study (VIGOR) in which the safety and efficacy of rofecoxib was compared with the safety/efficacy of an older product, Naproxen. This study found that patients treated with rofecoxib had an increased risk of heart disease compared with patients treated with Naproxen. Within the company, this finding raised further concerns relating to the underlying pharmacodynamic mechanism, but these were not clearly conveyed to the public.

A second trial ('APPROVe'), in which the potential positive therapeutic effects for a different indication (treatment in patients with GI-polyps) was studied, found clearer indications of cardiovascular problems. Merck withdrew rofecoxib from the market in September 2004, informing the authorities, who had not been notified of problems earlier, on that same day.

The findings with rofecoxib had consequences for all medications in the same class, but also for products that had been on the market for decades. The Vioxx affair was the starting point for a thorough analysis by the Institute of Medicine, a US institution, on the ways in which pharmacovigilance should be performed in the US.

Rosiglitazone (Avandia) – an unfinished puzzle

At the time of writing, the discussion around the risk–benefit of rosiglitazone is ongoing. Rosiglitazone (Avandia) is a medicinal product approved in 1999 for the treatment of non-insulin dependent diabetes (diabetes type 2). Rosiglitazone is primarily an insulin-sensitiser which acts through sensitising the peripheral tissues for body-own insulin produced. Rosiglitazone reduces the plasma glucose levels (the amount of sugar in the blood) and the glucose formation by the liver, as well as improving glucose tolerance in patients with diabetes mellitus type 2. Rosiglitazone is generally well-tolerated and has, thanks to its mechanism of action, a limited risk of hypoglycaemia (too strong a decrease of sugar levels). Because of the complementary mechanism of action (additional to the existing oral anti-diabetics medicines), important decreases of HbA1c occur. HbA1c is a compound often measured in blood which indicates the average blood sugar level. In Europe, the use of rosiglitazone is currently limited to the concomitant treatment with metformin and sulphonylurea derivatives, whereas in the US it may also be used as a stand-alone medication. In addition, in the US it may also be used in combination with insulin, unlike in the EU, where this is not recommended.

In a recently completed meta-analysis (an evaluation of multiple studies) of studies, mainly conducted in the US, an increased risk was found for heart attacks and the occurrence of heart failure in connection with the use of rosiglitazone. The interpretation of these findings was difficult, as the indications (as described earlier) and the contraindications differed between the US and Europe. In the EU, even at the beginning of the assessment of the Avandia dossier, there were concerns regarding the retention of fluids and the resulting risk of heart failure, which was listed in the product information. Heart failure in the EU is a contraindication, and the product may not be used in patients with this disease. In the US, a more recent warning regarding the occurrence of heart failure was published, and the recommendation not to use rosiglitazone in patients with heart failure was included in the US product information in August 2007. In a more recent publication, the EMA stated that the risk–benefit balance is still positive, although a warning was added for patients with ischaemic heart disease. A similar warning was also added to the US patient information. The question that remains is, in what way does pioglitazone, a member of the same thiazolidin derivatives class, have a different risk profile with regard to ischaemic heart disease, as there is no difference with regard to the risk of the occurrence of heart failure.

Conclusion

In summary, these events show that admitting a medicinal product to the market is not an endpoint, but the beginning of a new phase in the lifecycle of a product. It is paramount to monitor a medicine closely so that new insights into the risk–benefit balance are detected early, and measures can be taken. These events also show that the relatively new field of pharmacovigilance is an evolving specialty, and all stakeholders are looking for a way to organise the sources of information to get the greatest benefit from it, and to safeguard public health as well as possible. It is now widely accepted that the safety of any medicinal product is only partly known at the time the new product comes onto the market, and that the risk–benefit balance is more clearly determined with everyday use. Formats to optimise post-marketing information have been discussed in the literature and offer opportunities for the future and challenges for everyone working in pharmacovigilance (see Figure 3).

Frits Lekkerkerker emphasised the importance of pharmacovigilance in an interview in a Dutch pharmaceutical periodical.[2] He also pointed out its strengthened position in the new Dutch Medicines Act which came into effect in July 2007. This law gives priority to the interests of patients. Every effort must be made to prevent and limit harmful effects in

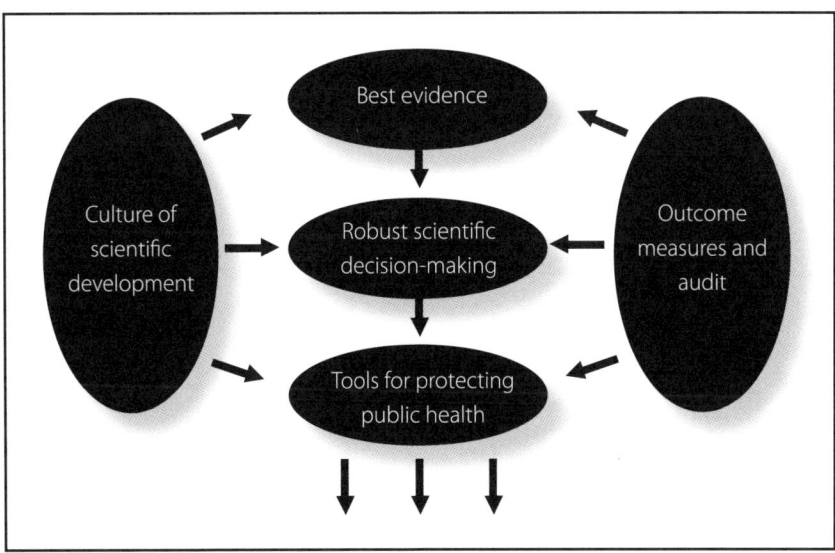

Figure 3: Measurable performance in terms of public health benefit.

vulnerable patients. This requires intensive cooperation among professionals, registration authorities, universities, pharmaceutical companies and the media, to increase information on the balance between risk and benefit, and to convey this information appropriately to the public, and to further improve patient care. New European legislation offers numerous possibilities, and much can be expected from the political efforts being carried out in Europe. Trust is essential, but unfortunately recent developments have not promoted this. A renewed effort is necessary to restore this trust and to give new developments a chance.

References

[1] *AEC Directive 65/65.*
[2] *Pharmaceutisch Weekblad, 13 mei 2005.*

Bibliography

Fraunhofer Report, January 2006.
Institute of Medicine, 'The future of Drug Safety', September 2006.
H M Krumholz, J L Ross, A H Presler, D S Egilman. 'What have we learnt from Vioxx?' BMJ 2007; 334:120-3.
S Nissen, K Wolski. 'Effect of Rosiglitazone on the Risk of Myocardial Infarction an Cardiovascular Death', NEJM, 2007; 356.
D Psaty. 'Protecting the Health of the Public Institute of Medicine Recommendations on Drug Safety', NEJM 2006; 355; 17; 1753-55.
P Walter, S Evans. 'A model for the future conduct of Pharmacovigilance', Pharmaco-epidemiology and Drug Safety 2003; 12/17-29.

11

The pharmaceutical industry and the MEB – friend or foe?

by Fred Schobben

The relationship between the MEB and the pharmaceutical industry is a strange one. Both strive to provide safe and effective medicines, yet their interests seem to differ.

The MEB, as independent organisation, grants MAs on behalf of the government. It does so only after evaluating the balance between risk and benefit and, as has been noted elsewhere, it will only grant an MA if it is convinced that the benefits outweigh the risks for patients.

The pharmaceutical industry, on the other hand, is commercially active and companies try to regain their high investments from the development of new medicinal products as quickly as possible. The registration procedure forms a significant hurdle in this process.

It also seems as if the pharmaceutical industry is the commissioner of the MEB, since it actually finances the agency while the MEB judges the industry's activities, from the development of new medicines to the safety monitoring of existing medicinal products.

In previous years the MEB also organised regular information days, together with Nefarma, the Dutch organisation of manufacturers of innovative medicinal products, to recruit new people to the field. This did not contribute to the image of an independent organisation that the MEB is supposed to be. Some people have even openly questioned whether the MEB is indeed independent.

In an article in a professional publication in 2006, it was stated: 'There are relationships between registration authorities and the pharmaceutical industry which are not always clear. The procedures and evaluation mechanisms are not well enough known. Warranty of the independence of the authorities and scientific personnel is not sufficiently clear. The direct financial dependence on the pharmaceutical industry, by the industry paying for its MAs, creates an aura of dependence'.[1]

An important part of this criticism is dealt with in the new European legislation regarding transparency. A good relationship between the registration authorities and the industry is essential however. Only when information is exchanged adequately can good medicinal products become available to the public as quickly and safely as possible.

There are sufficient safeguards to guarantee that the main task of the MEB – providing the public with effective and safe medicinal products – is met. Members of the MEB are questioned annually about their relationships with the industry. Possible conflicts of interest are announced on the MEB's website.[2] Attempts by the industry to influence members of the MEB are strongly denounced. Financial interests barely play a role, as the fees charged for the application and the maintenance of the registration are determined by law, and do not depend on the outcome of the decision on the application. The activities to be performed during the review procedure, covered by this fee, are determined by national or European regulation. The joint information sessions organised by the MEB and the Nefarma have been discontinued.

The battle for experts

Of course, the pharmaceutical industry tries to present its products in the best possible light. The MEB requires detailed information so that it can scrutinise the data on the new medicinal product. Claims by the industry need to be well-founded in order to be included in the SmPC. This information also forms the basis for the claims that can be made in promotional material.

The MEB employs a broad range of experts to thoroughly evaluate each application. If necessary, these experts have access to a pool of outside specialists who can be consulted on particular issues. However, following any consultation, the MEB will always make its decisions independently. It is true, however, that the MEB will recruit its scientific advisers from the same pool of experts that the pharmaceutical industry does: the creation of a registration dossier and its evaluation require the same knowledge. Payment will likely be better in the industry than at the agency, and often experts go from the MEB to the industry. However, not everyone feels comfortable in the commercial world, and the reverse is possible too!

Conflicts

There are often conflicts between the MEB and the industry when companies apply for an MA for a new product or for an authorisation for a new therapeutic indication for an existing product. The company wants to market the product as soon as possible, but the MEB may often consider the application premature. Companies assume that the missing data will become available during the application process and can be submitted at a later date. But the evaluation of such dossiers is more cumbersome than a dossier that is complete when it is initially submitted. This understandable behaviour by the industry sometimes leads to unnecessary irritation on both sides, but this route also usually leads to the required well-founded evaluation of the data.

Pharmacovigilance also causes conflicts. According to the MEB, the industry should put more effort into conducting a timely fulfilment of its pharmacovigilance responsibilities. After all, the safety of patients is at stake!

If the MEB seriously doubts the reliability of the provided data, it asks the Health Inspectorate to inspect the data locally or even to inspect the entire organisation of clinical trials by the company. If the result is that certain data are found to be insufficiently reliable, this can lead to a rejection or cancellation of an application, which does not improve relations between the industry and the MEB.

In the case of an imminent rejection of an application of a product or new indication, hearings will be held between the MEB and the company involved. This can also happen if important data come to light for an existing registration. The company then brings in lawyers and international experts to prove its case. This sometimes leads to interesting scientific or legal debates. After the meeting, the company submits its arguments again in writing. The MEB will then re-evaluate the data. The initial decision is sometimes reversed if the company's case is supported.

The 'battle' between the MEB and the industry is often about commas in PILs and SmPCs. The industry likes to show positive claims or extensive indications; the MEB only wants to include proven effects and relevant data. There are often several drafts before the final text is approved.

A known problem is the description of side-effects. The industry wants to protect itself from claims, while the MEB only wants to mention the information that is relevant for the physician and the patient. The discussion usually ends with the conclusion that the drug developer cannot be kept from mentioning an observed effect in the SmPC.

A company sometimes sues the MEB in order to get more information from the competitors registration dossier disclosed, referring to the Freedom of Information Act. When the MEB denies such a request, the judge will usually do the same. This indicates that there are still economic interests that need to be respected. It often concerns data on the exact composition, or the preparation, of a medicinal product and information on the status of the MA. However, the MEB believes that all the information relevant to the correct use of a medicinal product needs to be known to the patient and the physician. Companies are concerned about releasing information that could be of interest to their competitors, or that might have a negative effect on their ranking in the financial market.

The MEB is also sometimes sued when it has decided to grant an MA. In such cases, the developer of an innovative product is generally trying to keep generic products from the market. Seldom is the industry found to be in the right, but it leads to a delay in the implementation of the decision to market the product, which is usually beneficial for the plaintiff.

Consultation

During the development of a new product, a company can ask the MEB for advice about the course it wants to follow. This usually happens once, and typical questions include: 'Are there any gaps in the documentation', or 'Could this specific route lead to a certain indication description?' The advice does not guarantee a final positive decision, but it can be instructive for companies.

The MEB consults four times a year with branch organisations from the pharmaceutical industry. The relationships in these meetings differ because these consultations do not concern specific products. Even so, the industry's interests do differ. Companies producing generic products have different interests from innovator companies. Some measures will give more protection to the original product than the generic. Companies concentrating on parallel imports (where a legitimate medicinal product is imported without the permission of the drug producer, generally because the imported drug is cheaper in the exporting country and so a profit can be made following importation) do have other interests. During these quarterly meetings, implementation of new rules and regulations are discussed and the MEB gives information about projects that it is working on. The parties reach agreements on streamlining and unification, and on trust and transparency. These decisions are not laws and cannot be enforced to individual companies, but they do contribute to progress.

An example of this was some companies' practice of withdrawing an application if it was thought that a denial was pending. Because the application was withdrawn before the official decision, it meant the MEB was unable to give its arguments for refusing the application, even when publication of these arguments could be in the public interest. Thanks to a 'gentleman's agreement' reached in this particular consultation, this information can now be made public.

There is international cooperation in the development of European regulation and in the ICH. Here, guidelines are developed by different registration authorities and concept regulations are sent to the industry.[3] The final text, however, is determined by the authorities.

Industry *vs* the MEB

In general, the industry appears to regard the MEB as annoying but fair. The MEB, on the other hand, sees the industry more often as keepers of their own possessions than as protectors of the patient. The relationship can best be described as respectful but with a dose of suspicion. This seems like a healthy attitude.

References

[1] C Overdijk. *'De evolutie van de rol van de farmceutische industrie in de gezondheidszorg', Geneesmiddelenbulletin 2006;40;111-116.*
[2] *www.cbg-meb.nl/nl.overcbg*
[3] *www.ch.org*

12

The physician, the pharmacist and the MEB

by Arno Hoes

The MEB's role of granting MAs for medicinal products, withdrawing products if there is reason to do so, and determining the delivery status of products on the market in the Netherlands, sometimes leads to lengthy and heated debates – for example, the debate on the delivery status of emergency contraceptives (the 'morning-after pill'). The MEB is also involved in the daily clinical and pharmaceutical practice, as medicinal products are crucial to patient care.

Evidence-based medicine and evidence-based regulatory practice

In the scientific evaluation of medicinal products, the risk–safety balance takes centre stage. This scientific evaluation requires a critical evaluation of all available scientific evidence of benefits and side-effects of the medicine in the category of patients for whom it is intended. This forms the basis of evidence-based medicine, that is, daily use based on all available scientific knowledge – a key part of the decision-making process of the MEB, alongside its access to other important tools of evidence-based medicine such as data from the randomised trial or the meta-analysis. If put this way, you could summarise the task of the MEB as evidence-based regulatory practice.

However, everyday clinical practice is not always determined by available evidence. Many interventions are not yet proven to have a scientific foundation. This can happen because, for example, the medicinal product was marketed before the acceptance of randomised trials as the gold standard in proving the efficacy of a medicinal product.

A randomised trial is an experiment in which a group of patients with a certain illness is studied, with some of them receiving the investigational medicinal product and the others receiving a placebo. The selection of the treatment, ie, active or placebo, is determined randomly.

The outcome of the first formal randomised trial was published in 1948 in the British Medical Journal. It was a study into the effect of the antibiotic streptomycin in patients with pulmonary tuberculosis[1] Evidence-based medicine cannot be considered cookbook medicine. It is not just evidence that is important – the experience of the physician and the preferences of the patient must also be taken into account. If research proves that an antibiotic is highly effective for treating ear infections in very young children, the physician has to determine with the parent if the positive effect of the medication outweighs the risk of diarrhoea.[2] The evidence, if available, is important, but not the sole determination in the decision to prescribe the medicine.

In the evidence-based regulatory practice of the MEB, other scientific factors play a role, albeit that the scientific factors of evidence-based medicine are the most important. It is hard to imagine discussions on the delivery status of an emergency contraceptive based solely on scientific arguments. Solid state-of-the-art evidence is difficult to imagine. There will never be a randomised trial in which some women, living in some regions, will be able to get their morning-after pill by prescription only, while other women in other regions will be able to buy the medication over the counter. Subsequently, it would need to be measured which method of intervention has the most positive effect in avoiding abortions, now or next year. As with evidence-based medicine, in evidence-based regulatory practice one has to take account of the preferences of the patient and clinical experience, along with scientific evidence. This means that the MEB needs to understand and take into account daily clinical practice as it makes its decisions.

The MEB and daily practice

An important way to ensure that the MEB stays is touch with everyday clinical practice is to recruit members who are working in clinical, pharmaceutical, or scientific fields. Many MEB employees do indeed work in those fields, besides their part-time post at the MEB. However, it is not possible to have all relevant clinical and scientific expertise in-house. To fill these voids, the MEB can hire outside experts on an ad hoc basis, or in a more formal setting (see Chapter 10). In addition, these experts can be involved in discussions at the EMA meetings, when a decision is made about the registration or withdrawal of a medicinal product in the EU. There are more than 200 Dutch experts registered with the EMA, providing a great diversity of expertise, and they can act in an advisory role for both the EMA and the MEB

Paediatric medicines: an example of intensive collaboration

Many medicinal products prescribed for children have not or have barely been tested in children. It was long believed that it was irresponsible to have children participate in randomised trials, as this would subject this vulnerable group of patients to possible harmful effects of medications. Children are not guinea pigs. Also, the knowledge that children cannot usually make well-informed decisions about participation in a trial, but that the parent or guardian must decide for them, has played a role in this decision. The lack of evidence of efficacy and side-effects leads, however, to a situation where medicines are being used incorrectly in children or are being withheld without cause. Recently, the notion has developed that it is better to have a small group of children participate in a well-conducted experiment in order to be able to measure the effects of a medicinal product reliably and securely. Not to do this can lead to a situation where physicians prescribe medications that are not evidence-based on a much wider scale. Many diseases occurring in children need to be treated, and it is better if interventions are prescribed using evidence-based information.

In 2007, the Regulation on Medicinal Products for Paediatric Use[3] was enacted and the PDCO was founded. This committee consists of paediatricians and other experts who play a central role in the EMA when evaluating medicines for use in children. One of the determinations that they decide is the necessity of using children when testing a particular medicinal product – there is no point, for example, in testing a medication for geriatric use, as the product would never be indicated for use in children.

These developments will eventually lead to the situation where medicines that will be prescribed to children will have been tested in children, and this will also promote the development of special paediatric medicinal products and formulations. The industry is 'rewarded' for such testing with an extra six months of patent protection if research has been done in children.

Parallel to these developments in Europe, the Netherlands also set up a group comprising experts in pharmacotherapy in children. As of February 2006, this group (Klankbord Kinderartsen) advises on registration of medicinal products for children. They also act as peer reviewers for Dutch reports that are submitted in Europe, and as experts in the Netherlands and the UK. The creation of a separate expert group for children, consisting of practitioners in the field, illustrates the importance of involving practical experience in the work of the MEB.

Communications with physicians and pharmacists

The MEB seeks to inform physicians and pharmacists of the most important developments related to the registration and safety of medicinal products, and to share its knowledge with these professionals. It strives for maximum transparency, although there are legal limits. Within these limits, however, the MEB's communication with physicians and pharmacists needs to be optimised. It is to be hoped that all limits will eventually be removed, so that full transparency can be achieved. The MEB's recently updated website can contribute to this effort.

The MEB also reports on new developments on its website. For example, its homepage on 22 March 2008 reported safety information on bortezomib (Velcade) and natalizumab (Tysabri) and described the MEB's position on antidepressants following a recent meta-analysis which stated that the efficacy of newer antidepressants was inferior. In cases of acute problems with the safety of a medicinal product, letters to physicians and pharmacists form an important additional source of communication. These letters, now known as Direct Healthcare Professional Communications (DHPCs), but formerly called 'dear doctor letters', are sent out by the pharmaceutical companies themselves (the registration holders of the suspect products), as instructed by the MEB or the IGZ. The MEB also publishes articles in Dutch professional periodicals.

Do practitioners know the MEB?

Considering the role that the MEB plays in communicating with and advising physicians and pharmacists, the question remains as to the extent that healthcare professionals are aware of the function of the MEB. To establish this, pharmacists and physicians in the northern and eastern parts of the Netherlands were polled between February 2007 and February 2008. Our findings revealed that only 30% of respondents knew the meaning of the acronym MEB, and another 20% knew it was a committee dealing with registrations of medicinal products. It was remarkable that more people were familiar with the acronym 'FDA' (the Food and Drug Administration) – the MEB's US counterpart – than with either the MEB's acronym or Europe's medicines regulator, the EMA.

Clearly, the MEB needs to have scientific expertise as well as knowledge about everyday clinical practice in order to enable evidence-based regulatory practice. It obtains this knowledge by selecting its members from professionals who work part-time in clinical or scientific fields, and by involving formal or ad hoc groups of experts in its decision-making. Communication with physicians and pharmacists through its website, DHPCs and publications in professional periodicals are of increasing importance.

References

[1] *Medical Research Council: 'Streptomycin treatment of pulmonary tuberculosis', BMJ 1948 2:769-82.*

[2] *M M Rovers, P Glasziou, C L Appelman, P Burke, D P McCormick, R A Damoiseaux, I Gaboury, P Little, A W Hoes. 'Antibiotics for acute otitis media, a meta-analysis with individual patient data', Lancet 2006; 368: 1429-35.*

[3] *Regulation 1901/2006 EU.*

13

Informing and cooperating with patient and consumer organisations

by Jan Schellens

This chapter provides a brief summary of some key points detailed earlier in this book in relation to the MEB's aims, and its remit in working with patients and patient/consumer organisations.

As the MEB works on behalf of the patient, it is logical that patient and consumer organisations are closely involved in the process of registering medicinal products. It is also important that they are informed of new developments, such as new safety information that becomes available following registration, once a medicine is in everyday use in a 'real world' setting.

Transparency

In recent years the MEB has decided that the registration procedure should be as transparent as possible. This has not always been the case, as, under pressure from the pharmaceutical industry, all data that the MEB received were previously kept secret. However, this was found to be against the public interest, which requires transparency. This means that anyone can be informed of new medicinal products as they come onto the market, and be advised, for example, of a medication's possible benefits and side-effects, and of which patient populations (if any) might have special risk factors when using the product.

Under the MEB's remit to advise and inform patients, it considers that all written information should be available in everyday language that is comprehensible to laymen. Patients, physicians and pharmacists should also have access to information on medications for which an application for marketing authorisation has been denied. All of this information is available on the MEB's website.

MEB initiatives

To inform patients as fully as possible, the MEB has taken a number of initiatives, including being closely involved in the founding of the 'EMA/CPMP working group with patient organisations' in 2002.

Some of the recommendations this group has made are:
● To clarify the registration process, and the distribution of information about this process
● To find ways to improve product information and pharmacovigilance
● To increase cooperation between patient organisations and the EMA.

Nationally, the MEB has taken the initiative in consulting with Dutch patient organisations. These organisations meet twice a year with the head of the MEB, and the intention is to increase their frequency to quarterly meetings.

The MEB listens to patient organisations

Patient groups are being asked their opinion on repeat prescriptions and the contents and readability (in terms of comprehension) of PILs. Patient organisations and consumer organisations are also consulted about OTC medicines and products that are used in children.

To make this a workable process, there are guidelines on which groups are eligible to participate in these consultations. These can be general umbrella organisations or organisations representing specific conditions such as cancer, diabetes, Alzheimer's, and so on. They need to be registered organisations and represent Dutch patients and consumers.

Improving contact with patients

An important development in patient contact is the ability for patients to report side-effects. In the Netherlands, this can be done at Lareb, which reports back to the MEB. As noted in earlier chapters, patients can now report adverse events directly to Lareb on its website (www.lareb.nl/melden/patient.asp). The Netherlands is the first country to offer such a reporting system to its population and, thus far, the experiences have been positive, with patients keen to contribute actively to increasing the safety of medicinal products.

So what does the future hold? It is expected that contact between the MEB and patient and consumer organisations will increase. The MEB is fully dedicated to this consultation process. Patient and consumer organisations are encouraged to participate actively. This collaboration is progressing well, and will lead to improvements in the information given to patients/consumers, improvements in the safety of medicinal products, and the more rational use of medicines.

14

Paediatric medicines and the MEB

by Jan Taminiau and Henk van den Berg

As highlighted in Chapter 12, most medicinal products prescribed for children have not been researched in children. This was previously deemed unnecessary because drug developers apply for MAs for their chosen indications and their chosen age groups. Applying for registration for a product's use in children was considered unrealistic, partly because research in children is cumbersome and expensive, and partly because of the ethical issues involved in testing paediatric populations.

However, accidents have happened because 'adult' medicines have been given to children. A well-known example is the death of children following the use of an antibiotic (sulphanilamide) elixir, using diethylene glycol (antifreeze), which created a toxic formulation. Unborn children have also been at risk, for example with the well-known thalidomide affair discussed in earlier chapters.

Medicines are expected to have a healing effect, but many that are useful in adults can be toxic in children. This is because children's metabolism is different from adults, with products being distributed differently in the body, or discharged differently through urine, for instance.

Examples of this are benzodiazepines, which have a limited effect in children, and the extreme sensitivity of newborns to opiates. As a result of reduced activity of metabolic enzymes, some drugs (such as cisapride, an antiemetic) can be dangerous when used in young children, due to the inactivity of CYP 3A4 – an enzyme in the liver involved with the metabolism of many medicines.

In summary, there are differences between young children and adults with regard to absorption, distribution, metabolism and elimination (ADME). Because of this unpredictability, additional research is required, and simple extrapolation from data obtained in adults is not possible. This research in children needs to include ADME from the child's body. Attention should also be paid to any undesirable effects of the medicinal product on the maturation of the body and the ripening of organs. The location where the medicinal product exerts its pharmacological effect might not be developed yet, or the target may have a different expression in children. These are all reasons to research efficacy and side-effects of use of a medicinal product in children.

It is not just the active ingredient that can be a cause for concern; the excipients can also pose a risk. Because of the intended efficacy and medical necessity, medications must be prescribed for sick children. One study[1] found that 48% of medications used in a Dutch prenatal intensive care unit were unlicensed, and an additional 18% were prescribed off-label (ie, prescribed for a condition other than the therapeutic indication and/or age group approved by regulators). In general practice, the numbers are roughly the same.

The situation in the Netherlands is the same as in other European countries, and countries like the US and Australia. More worryingly, many physicians do not know if a medicinal product is registered for the specific indication or age group.

As noted earlier, there are ethical reasons for not conducting research in children. It can be seen as irresponsible to use children as 'guinea pigs' without them being able to decide to participate for themselves. The burden (from injections, pain, or long-term restriction of mobility) could also be considered unethical. On the other hand, it has been argued that because of the differences in ADME between adults and children, it is irresponsible to prescribe medicinal products to children based on the extrapolation of data from testing in adults.

In this atmosphere, paediatric legislation (comprising Regulation (EC) No 1901/2006 and the amending Regulation (EC) No 1902/2006) came into force on 26 January 2007, requiring medicines to be researched in children. As a direct result of this, the Dutch Centre of Pharmacotherapy in Children (NKFK) was founded. It is intended to be the source of information for physicians. It also publishes a Paediatric Formulary, which gives guidelines for prescribing medicines to children based on the best evidence available. Another organisation that was founded was the Dutch Medicines Research Network, MCRN, which plays a coordinating role in all paediatric research in the Netherlands.

The UK, Germany, Austria and Finland already have similar centres, and other countries will follow. These national networks, as required by the Directive, will be linked in to an umbrella organisation in which the EMA will also be involved.

The most important contributions to the responsible prescribing of medicinal products for children are the new registration procedures. The paediatric regulation states that all new registrations after January 2009 must have the approval of the EMA's Paediatric Committee (PDCO). To get approval, a research plan (known as a paediatric investigation plan, or PIP) in which the medicine is trialled in children must be submitted. For indications that do not or seldom incur in children, a waiver can be granted. In cases where the producer of the medicinal product wants to market the product for use in adults before research in children is completed, a deferral can be issued.

When a manufacturer markets a product, it is given two years of market exclusivity. In the case of an orphan drug (see Chapter 17) this period is ten years. In cases where the paediatric research has been executed correctly, according to the approved PIP, six months or two years' additional marketing exclusivity is granted. In instances where a product is off-patent and a new dosage form or new therapeutic indication is investigated according to an approved PIP, ten years data protection or exclusivity will be awarded (the so-called Paediatric Use Marketing Authorisation (PUMA)). During this time the manufacturer has a chance to regain its additional development costs. In the US, similar legislation has been in force for some time. This legislation has not just given producers additional financial gain, but also increased the knowledge of the effects of medicinal products on different age groups.

New medicinal products

What changes did the new regulation create in the development and use of new medicinal products in children? It is logical to first test the efficacy and safety of new medicinal products in adults. However, this means that a medicine will be evaluated for use in children several years later, after it has been used for some time in adult populations, by which time the drug developer may not be interested in conducting additional testing. Because of this, it is preferable to see if it is possible to test a medicinal product simultaneously in adults and in children, assuming that there is a need for an indication for use in children.

However, this raises several questions: Are there enough therapies already available among current medicinal products? Can toxicological research in animals give an indication of the safety of the medicine for young organ systems, and can such research determine that there will be no negative effects on mental development and neurological growth in humans? As side-effects can prove different both in adult humans and in children when compared with animal research, a strong system of pharmacovigilance is an absolute necessity.

Registered medicines with market exclusivity

Before market exclusivity for a particular medicinal product ends, a producer can extend it by conducting the necessary research in children at this time. Many companies will weigh the cost of such research against the gains of an additional six months of exclusivity.

Old medicinal products

Research on old medicines to ascertain their efficacy and safety when used in children has a long way to go. Many older products have insufficient data, or data are missing altogether. To promote research in this category of products, a priority list has been created. This list comprises products for which there is great need, often because there are few or no other medicines for this indication, and the indication is fairly common. Alternatively, it may be a medicinal product for a less common indication but with a need for additional information for clarification on aspects of an existing medicine, usually a generic. Because of the low price of these older or generic products, companies often do not have the funds to finance the additional research. To resolve this problem, the EU has made funds available to research these generic medicinal products. It is possible that a medicine's safety will be a reason for further research under the new pharmacovigilance system being created in Europe.

Stipulations for research with children as study subjects

Regulations with regard to registration are insufficient to be used alone as a guide to good research. Research methods for trials in children need to be described, and need to be related to the type of disease and specific requirements for children. Objective, measurable and reproducible goals for studies need to be defined. Formulations appropriate for child administration need to be developed. To protect the child and to ensure they follow Good Paediatric Practice (GPP), many guidelines will be created specifically for different indications to enable responsible and reproducible research.

The role of the MEB

For many years, the MEB has been involved in numerous initiatives relating to the use of medicinal products in children. It set up a study group comprising paediatricians, pharmacists and pharmacologists with special expertise with children. With the enactment of the European regulation, the MEB has played an important role and, in the ensuing Paediatric Committee, the Dutch representatives are among the most active members.

To sum up, the use of medicinal products by children received very little attention on the legislative stage until recently. This is changing rapidly. Existing gaps will be filled and, for new registrations, testing in children is now mandatory (where applicable). Much needs to be done in the coming years, but these actions will undoubtedly lead to better medicines for children.

References

[1] *A survey on the use of off-label and unlicensed drugs in a Dutch children's hospital. G W Jong, A G Vulto, M de Hoog, K J Schimmel, D Tibboel, J N van den Anker. Pediatrics, 2001 Nov;108(5):1089-93.*

15

Evaluating 'strange' medicines

by Emiel van Galen

Strange feelings scare. Strange things also arouse curiosity. The MEB's function is to weigh up the benefit–risk balance of any medicinal product, including those that are not primarily 'evidence-based', such as homeopathic, herbal and anthroposophic medicinal products.

The MEB is very precise in all its evaluations, but it still has its critics. At times the agency has been accused of being too far removed from the way in which medicines are used in daily life. Some critics have said that the MEB stares blindly at an SmPC but barely notices, and pays too little attention to, the way a product is used in the real world. [1]

There is a certain amount of conflict, too, between medical professionals who dispense 'alternative' medicines [2] and those who take the pharmacological-medical approach to proof of efficacy based on scientific principles, and a society in which alternative products and 'strange' medicines are still prominently present.

The MEB, in the midst of these criticisms and conflicts, has been tasked with evaluating alternative medicines since 1997. The EU determined more than a decade ago that these products should be regulated, partly because of the increasing number of people who use them, and partly because any potential negative effects needed to be brought to light.

The legal function of a competent authority is to guarantee the safe use of medicinal products. An MEB evaluation focuses on the contents of the bottles, but the question remains – is it possible to use the same criteria that apply to 'evidence-based' medicines for 'alternative' medicinal products? With such products, 'old' does not automatically mean outdated, and many people value these centuries-old treatments.

Evaluation and registration of these types of medicines has been a slow process until now. In Europe, the MEB was quickly seen as a very strict evaluator, but at least its evaluation criteria were clear. Within the EU Directive, a simplified evaluation model was defined that was supposed to handle the 'strange proofs' of efficacy and evaluate these medicines on their own merits. The general concept introduced in European legislation pays respect to 'traditional use'.

Traditional use

Alternative methods of treatment use medicinal products with a long tradition. These medicines have proved themselves through longstanding use and historic experience, and are often accepted as effective by both practitioners and users, even without scientific proof.

The MEB first evaluated traditional products using the rules for homeopathic products. Later, the agency also looked at other products that needed to be evaluated within the traditional settings in which they are used. These products required a separate system of evaluation criteria within the EU, even if they have been used daily in medical care in other parts of the world. Such treatments are based on therapeutic systems and philosophies that are far from the medical-scientific approach taken in Europe.

The producers of these medicines are not obliged to apply for the simplified procedures, for example for herbal medicines. However, producers can submit a complete dossier and apply for mutual recognition if they obtain a national registration fulfilling all requirements. They can even send a dossier to the European Medicines Agency, for central evaluation by the CHMP. This may be the only possible route for those indications for which the centralised procedure is mandatory. Herbal medicines are not exempt from this; if a herbal medicinal product claims to be effective in treating diabetes, it must be approved by the EMA, even if centuries of traditional use for diabetes can be proved. This is stated in the preamble to Directive 2004/24:

'Where the applicant can demonstrate by detailed references to published scientific literature that the constituent or the constituents of the medicinal product has or have a well-established medicinal use with recognised efficacy and an acceptable level of safety within the meaning of Directive 2001/83/EC, he/she should not be required to provide the results of preclinical tests or the results of clinical trials.' [3]

The foundation for registration based on tradition was not as a result of the fact that many medicinal products, primarily herbs, did not comply with the requirements for an MA, nor an authorisation based on accepted use. It was recognised in 2004 that several member states regulated these products through different procedures at national levels. This, of course, was detrimental to a harmonised EU market.

Traditional use as a concept seems to have been born of necessity. To achieve a harmonised market, longstanding traditional use of such products is taken as the starting point, following which requirements can be applied to check safety and quality.

The first Directive in this field, 92/73/EC, gave member states a simplified evaluation system for homeopathic medicines. Primary attention was given to pharmaceutical quality, together with an objective decision on the safety of the dilutions, and it was never assumed that the product would be safe simply because it was diluted. This procedure became known as the simplified procedure, which can only be used for homeopathic products that are administered orally or externally; for products that have no indication on the package or PIL; and are diluted at least 1:10,000 from the original ingredient. Now, ten years later, this simplified procedure has been implemented in all EU member states. It is the foundation for an almost harmonised evaluation and for regular European exchange of regulatory experiences. Mandatory registration for these homeopathic medicines is now a fact in the EU.

In 2000, a similar discussion began with regard to amending legislation so that it could apply to the registration of herbal medicinal products. This resulted in a simplified evaluation based, as with homeopathic products, on its traditional use. Such evaluation for homeopathic medicinal products was already *de facto* based on this concept; for herbal medicinal products it was legally established in 2004. The 2004 Directive is also the basis for the work of the Herbal Medicinal Products Committee (HMPC). Following this, further discussion began about the possible inclusion of categories of traditional medicinal products from China and India – parts of the world that get a lot of attention on many levels. Other categories of medicines within the EU which previously claimed not to have a place in the registration system are now asking for the same kinds of procedure.

European legislatures have discovered that defining an adapted evaluation based on characterising a special tradition for the use of unconventional medicinal products can be effective.

Herbal medicinal products

Herbal medicines still play an important role in many parts of the world. Even though there is a wealth of scientific knowledge about the effects of various herbs, this knowledge is literally scattered worldwide. Alongside the European traditions of herbal medicines or phytotherapy, (the study of the medicinal use of extracts of botanical origin), there is African herbal medicine, Unani medicine in Pakistan, traditional Chinese medicine (TCM), herbs with medicinal properties from the Amazon rainforests, and Ayurvedic herbal medicine from India, to name some the most important. Within the EMA's herbal committee, some local European specialities have also surfaced. In Latvia, for example, there is a vast store of knowledge on research that has been conducted with Siberian Ginseng *(Eleutherococcus senticosus)*.[4] Iceland has a wealth of information on Icelandic Moss *(Lichen islandicus)* and Norway has proved to be an expert on the herb commonly known as mullein or hedge-taper *(Verbascum thapsus)*.[5] The European Directive took European traditional medicine as a starting point; however, plants do not confine themselves to borders. The use of herbs in medical practice as described in the Directive goes further than just in the EU, or just in India, or just in the People's Republic of China. Scientific knowledge in this field can be found anywhere.

Fennel as a medicinal product

Fennel is the English name for *Foeniculum vulgare*, used as herbal tea. The material that supports traditional use has been evaluated by the EMA's Herbal Committee, and a monograph has been published[6] in which three traditional indications are mentioned:

- Traditional herbal medicinal product for symptomatic treatment of mild, spasmodic gastro-intestinal complaints including bloating and flatulence
- Traditional herbal medicinal product for symptomatic treatment of minor spasms, associated with menstrual periods
- Traditional herbal medicinal product used as an expectorant in cough, associated with common cold.

The monograph describes fennel's use as a domestic medicine, and its plausible effect is based on longstanding use and experience with the product as herbal tea in the EU. The monograph mentions the hypersensitivity for preparations using related plants, as a contraindication, and use by children under the age of four is discouraged as there is insufficient scientific research to evaluate safe use. Within Europe, however, there is much traditional knowledge on the use of this herbal product. In Dutch herbal literature, the herbal tea is recommended for babies as it tastes mild, and it persuades infants with diarrhoea to drink necessary liquids to ease digestive discomfort.[7] Germany and Austria have published similar information for use in their own countries. All these publications indicate European tradition, which does not equal scientific evidence for efficacy, and the discussion about proof of well-established use versus plausible effects based on proven traditional use is held continuously within the HMPC, and this dialogue will continue into the future.

Fennel is part of the European Pharmacopoeia with a monograph for the botanical material,[8] illustrating the herb's importance in the European tradition of medicinal products. It is also used in other parts of the world, where it appears that traditional use in those regions is based on the same plant and in a similar preparation.

Foeniculum vulgare is called Xiao hui xiang in traditional Chinese herbal medicine, and has similar indications, even though the concept of TCM is hard to compare with Western evidence-based medicine. A monograph for Xiao hui xiang is included in the official Pharmacopoeia of the People's Republic of China.

Fennel is called Razyana, or Samar, in Urdu, and in Pakistan it is also known as Saunf.[9] In Ayurvedic medicine it is known as Shatapushpa. The worldwide use of fennel is documented in Monographs on Selected Medicinal Plants, a WHO publication.[10]

As the MEB can make use of reviews performed by the HMPC and the WHO, the agency does not need to refer to a multitude of written sources, including sources that are of varying quality and date, in languages that are hard to understand, or describing traditions we can barely comprehend. For many herbal medicines there is much traditional scientific literature available, which can be the foundation for evaluation of quality and safety. Such evaluations make it easier to compare these traditional-use products with the evaluation of regular medicinal products with known active constituents.

Traditional Chinese medicinal products (TCM)

The scope of the term 'traditional Chinese medicinal products' needs to be limited to the part in which the MEB has a role. The evaluation of medicinal products from Chinese traditions often plays a distinct role in embracing the Peoples' Republic of China as a trade partner. TCM includes traditional Chinese medicinal products as well as treatments such as acupuncture and T'ai chi. In TCM, traditional diagnosis is based on completely different parameters, such as tongue diagnosis.

The evaluation of TCM products by EU member states is restricted to herbal products. Products with animal constituents are not included and are generally viewed with great suspicion in Europe. Even though the registration dossier does contain specific complex regulatory aspects, concerns that the MEB may have to evaluate bear bile or tiger bone are unfounded!

Closer to reality are the severe negative side-effects that have been associated with TCM products in the past decade. Martena[11] published an overview in 2007 of the results of an inspection of the presence of aristolochic acids in Chinese herbal products available in the Netherlands. By exchanging different aristolochic compounds in TCM medicines in 1993, severe cases of renal damage and carcinogenicity were reported and for this reason aristolochic compounds are not allowed without a previous evaluation and registration of the medicinal product. Despite the prohibition, 25 of the 68 researched products still showed traces of aristolochic acids.

The scope of evaluation of TCM products by the MEB is clearly defined as:

- Herbal medicinal products that contain one or more herbal compounds, one or more herbal preparations, or a combination thereof[12]

- Traditional products that contain animal excipients cannot be evaluated based on traditional use, according to the European Directive. The evaluation always relates to the packaged product, not the herbal material in its crude or prepared state

- Applications that can prove that all the requirements are met, including the requirement of traditional use, have to be submitted

- Herbs that contain known harmful compounds like aristolochic acids or pyrrolizidine alkaloids, or a herb such as *Ephedra vulgaris,* are prohibited from sale in their crude form, so their safety should always be established at registration as a medicinal product. Dangerous herbs are not prohibited in themselves, but their safety needs to be determined according to the appropriate guidelines

- The traditional medical use needs to be proven for at least 30 years, of which at least 15 years need to be within the borders of the current members of the EU

- For traditional herbal medicinal products, only those indications will be allowed which do not require the intervention or diagnosis of a medical professional, which in fact is self-medication (OTC).

The Chinese economy has developed rapidly in recent years, and so has its pharmaceutical industry. The thinking that the development of medicinal products will remain related for the most part to TCM seems to be incorrect. Although references are often made to the principles of TCM when in contact with Chinese producers, these are not usually related to the European system of traditional use that was introduced in 2004. Chinese producers present their plans to introduce modern Chinese herbal medicines based on TCM in Europe with great enthusiasm, and this is where the confusion starts. For some modern herbal medicines, scientific data from clinical research are available and considered to be the foundation of proof of efficacy. However, this is different from 'demonstrating plausible effect, based on long-term use and experience'. Herbal products sometimes have an active compound that carries the same plant name as a TCM compound, but which has been used in its modern form through advanced extraction methods. The Chinese pharmaceutical industry also produces traditional medicinal products for indications such as type-2 diabetes, hypertension, glaucoma, and the treatment of malignant diseases, all under the umbrella of TCM.

What contributes to the confusion is that, in Europe, the simplified vision of 'proof of efficacy' or 'based on traditional use' is paired with the normal standard level with regard to pharmaceutical quality. Tradition or not, the medicinal product needs to be of the highest standard. The question is, can all herbal medicines meet these standards?

A higher level of quality does not entitle a medicinal product to be dispensed for the more serious indications. In fact, the opposite is true. Herbal medicinal products need to comply with all European standards for quality, and there are plenty of these for herbal medicines, as well as the need to comply with the standards of the European Pharmacopoeia. Or, in the words of our herbal assessors : 'A constant, controllable quality is a first requisite for safety'. This definitely rings true for herbal medicines, wherever in the world they are prepared.

Homeopathic and anthroposophic medicinal products on the European market

The European Coalition on Homeopathic and Anthroposophic Medicinal Products (ECHAMP)[13] estimated the value of the European market of homeopathic and anthroposophic medicinal products in 2007 at €930 million. This market grew 60% between 1995 and 2005; it now makes up 7% of the total market for self-medications. The market share for homeopathic medicinal products alone is €810 million; the anthroposophic medicines have a €120 million share. Mandatory registration for all of these categories now applies throughout the EU.

Anthroposophic medicinal products

There is no definition for 'anthroposophic medicinal products' in European legislation, and its only mention is in the preamble to Directive 2001/83/EC:

'The anthroposophic medicinal products described in an official pharmacopoeia and prepared by a homeopathic method are to be treated, as regards registration and marketing authorisation, in the same way as homeopathic medicinal products.'[14]

In the Netherlands, anthroposophic medicinal products can only be sold if they are registered.[15] Anthroposophic medicines have been part of alternative medical care for a long time, and are being used by medical professionals in anthroposophic medicine.[16] Each pharmaceutical product used in a physician/patient relationship, in which both are aware of its therapeutic use based on anthroposophic principles, should be considered as an anthroposophic medicinal product, but, unfortunately, not by definition. Because there is no official definition for anthroposophic medicine or anthroposophic medicinal products in EU legislation, practitioners refer to the book by Rudolf Steiner for the origin of the anthroposophic approach to sickness and health,[17] and his collaboration with the Dutch physician Ita Wegman (c1920). Some materials used for anthroposophic products are included in the German homeopathic pharmacopoeia, but without specifying the 'anthroposophic background'.

In recent years, only 72 products have been registered in the Netherlands that can be considered as homeopathic medicinal products that are used according to anthroposophic philosophy. The future is hard to predict. Without the inclusion of anthroposophic methods and materials in an officially recognised pharmacopoeia, any adaptation of EU legislation will be complicated. Registration dossiers have been submitted and evaluated by the MEB for only a very small percentage of these medicinal products, but their use in primary medical care is much wider.

Registration of homeopathic medicines

In the Netherlands, the MEB has gained a wealth of regulatory experience during the past 15 years with the registration of homeopathic medicinal products. The end of 2009 saw 3,832 registered homeopathic medicines. All these products have been evaluated for consistent quality, and the safety of the dilutions has been verified. Physicians and industries in the homeopathic field argue that this number is still too low, and indicate they can no longer prescribe or distribute many of their products. Nevertheless, opponents of alternative healing methods say that every registered product is one too many. As noted at the beginning of this chapter, the MEB cannot do right by everyone at the same time.

In 1997, all homeopathic medicinal products that were on the market at the time had to be notified. There were more than 11,000. In this respect, in a decade of evaluation, the MEB has done well. During this timespan the MEB has had to defend its decision up to the highest courts when registration requests have been refused. The MEB was found to be right in every case, but it illustrates that the homeopathic field holds on strongly to a traditionally-created market reality.

The effects of homeopathy remain disputed, and give cause for occasional heavyweight and emotional debates in which parties can be poles apart. This is also seen in other EU member states. The controversy in homeopathy is that efficacy is expected from homeopathic medicines, but where there may be very little or no measurable amount of active compound in the final product, this raises the question: if there is nothing in there, how can it possibly have any effect?

Because the homeopathic tradition is primarily to be found in Europe, the first simplified legal procedure was written for homeopathic medicinal products. The most important goal was to guarantee good quality and safety. In hindsight, the procedure used then was already based on the concept of traditional use. Homeopathic use needs to be proven by practical use. The MEB's evaluation of many applications for these products – applying traditional principles for use while still looking at clear requirements for quality and safety – has had a tremendous effect, at least in the Netherlands. The MEB now has a proven record of evaluating unorthodox medicinal products, granting or denying registrations using a small group of specialist evaluators. With this experience, it is expected that the MEB will be able to evaluate other groups of medicinal products, even when their use is based on traditions that might initially seem strange.

References

[1] M Ivan Wolffers. 'CBG is de weg kwijt', Pharmaceutisch Weekblad, 2 November 2003.

[2] Margreet Vermeulen. 'Water en vuur', de Volkskrant, 29 November 2007 p.15.

[3] Directive 2004/24/EC (March 31 2004) regarding traditional herbal medicinal products.

[4] 'Reflection paper on the adaptogenic concept', (draft) EMEA/HMPC/102655/2007.

[5] Latvia is a member state of the EU, Iceland and Norway are member of the HMPC as observers, like Turkey and Croatia.

[6] A monograph of herbs is a scientific summary about the character of the herb and the data that are known about its use. The EMA Herbal Committee publishes Community Monographs with a content that is accepted by all member states. The WHO has also published monographs about the most important herbs that are used worldwide.

[7] J Van Hellemont. Fytotherapeutisch Compedium, tweede druk Houten, Bohn, Scheltema & Holkema 1988.

[8] A monograph in a pharmacopoeia like the European Pharmacopoeia (Ph Eur) describes the requirements of the quality of the basic compound, and does not contain any data on indication and use (compare reference 6).

[9] Khan Usmanghni. Indusyunic Medicine Traditional medicine of herbal origin in Pakistan , Karachi 1997.

[10] WHO monographs on Selected Medicinal Plants, Volume 3, Geneva: World Health Organization 2007.

[11] Martijn Martena e.a 'Enforcement of the ban on aristolochic acids in Chinese traditional herbal preparations on the Dutch market', Anal Bioanal. Chem.

[12] R M V Claessens. Tekst en toelichting Geneesmiddelen wet, Hoofdstuk 1 Begripsbepalingen en reikwijdte, artikel 1, eerste lid onder l.

[13] Homeopathic and Anthroposophic Medicine in Europe – Facts and Figures, second edition, Brussels; ECHAMP E/E/I/G/ 2007.

[14] Preamble 2001/83/EC article 22.

[15] Journaal Farmarecht, jaargang 2, nummer 5 (oktober 2007) , p.173.

[16] Gunver Sophia Kienle, Helmut and Hans-Ulrich Albonico. 'Anthroposophic Medicine Effectiveness, Utility, Costs, Safety', Stuttgart: Schattauer 2006.

[17] Rudolf Steiner. 'Geesteswetenschap en geneeskunde' (translated from German Geisteswissenschaft und Medizin) Zeist: Published by Vrij Geestesleven 1996.

6

Veterinary medicines – another world?

by Frank Verheijen

One of the most important things that men and animals have in common is their susceptibility to diseases. The risk of falling ill and the ability to cure is probably the most powerful way for Mother Nature to let the world be as it is. This might be a somewhat one-sided interpretation of Darwin's 'survival of the fittest', however, in evolutionary terms, only individuals that were able to survive attacks from micro-organisms reached the reproductive phase, and managed to give their healthy genes to their offspring. Also, the creativity to find enough food to survive, in combination with the ability to avoid being eaten by predators, increased the success rate for reaching the reproductive age. However, it became really interesting when some species, among them humans, realised that specific vegetation had healing properties.

By developing this experience instinctively and passing it on to the next generation, humans as well as other animals managed to avoid the strongest selection criteria: early death as a result of disease.

The reward for those creative individuals who used external aids to protect against illnesses was a higher life expectancy, and so an increased chance of producing offspring. At species level, however, this meant that not just the most physically fit survived and had offspring, but also those less physically fit but creative enough to use appropriate external aids. The survival of less 'fit' individuals does not by definition have to have a negative effect at species level. The success of humans as a species is the best proof of this.

While all animal species did not get further than establishing specific herbs in their menus instinctively, humans developed this knowledge by way of medicine men and the more-or-less accidental discovery of penicillin into a real pharmaceutical industry.

Humans did not develop their pharmaceutical knowledge solely for themselves, but also for animals and plants. By escaping a great part of the selection process through its powers of recuperation, the population increased to the extent that a new problem arose at population level: insufficient food. This new problem could only be resolved by developing structured, intense agricultural production systems.

The stimulation of European agriculture, initiated by the former Dutch EU commissioner Sicco Mansholt, turned out to be synonymous with the reality of monocultures and large stocks of animals. Certain rural areas developed into true 'veterinary metropoles' for chickens and pigs. Just like in cities with large populations, these concentrated areas are potential hotbeds of infection which can only be controlled with good hygiene, sophisticated vaccination programmes and the routine prophylactic and curative use of medicinal products. The human epidemiologist who thinks the spreading of illnesses in people is more complex because of international travel is wrong. Animals and plants are transported all over the world too.

The economic perspective

The high concentration of animal numbers increased the risk of infections and created a demand for veterinary medicines from an economic point of view. One of the world's largest companies producing veterinary medicines is a spin-off from a company producing animal feed. Sick animals eat less, which is bad for the feed business.

In modern animal husbandry, the economic arguments for using veterinary medicines are stronger than ever. In the past, a farmer had a small farm with different agricultural crops, 20 cows with names of his wife and daughters, and a few dozen chickens in the farmyard. Nowadays the agricultural entrepreneur manages a dairy farm, poultry farm or high-rise pig farm. The red-and-white Daisy 6 with her nice character and Cindy 11 with her beautiful blaze are condemned to an existence as rare traditional cow breeds.

Modern dairy farms use only high productive cows with Holstein-Friesian blood, all offspring of a few genetically closely related top sires. The most successful Dutch sire Sunny Boy had a progeny of more than one million calves. The farmer can only recognise his animals by the numbers on the ear tags. The computer automatically records the daily milk yield and balances the feeding of concentrated feed to optimise individual production. The most highly productive cows produce more than 10,000 kg of milk per year. During a large part of the lactation period, the animals suffer from a negative energy balance resulting in a higher susceptibility for mastitis and other infections. Chickens are moved from the farmyard into very large henhouses with sometimes more than 100,000 animals. From the same ancestor, totally different chicken breeds are created by selective breeding. Laying hens weigh around 1,500-1,700 grams and produce more than 300 eggs of 55-60 grams per year (this is in total ten times their own body weight). Broilers (meat production) grow from a lovely one-day old chicken weighing less than 50 grams to a slaughter weight of about 2.3 kilograms in less than six weeks. At a certain age, pigs grow more than 800 grams per day. Due to the competition at world market level, the profit for the farmer is limited to a few cents per litre of milk, egg or kilogram of meat. Only high numbers of animals per farm make it possible to earn a decent family income.

Animals have become a production tool with which the farmer tries to generate his income as efficiently as possible. For the farmer, the veterinary medicinal product is a management tool to optimise animal production. All costs for medicines directly influence the family income. Pet owners are also directly confronted with the costs of treatment. This cost awareness at micro-level is completely different from the decision model for prescribing medicines by a family doctor. The physician prescribes the best (most appropriate) medicine for his customer (the patient) and the costs are usually covered at a macro-level by public health budgets.

The strong emphasis on cost–benefit analysis is applicable to the entire veterinary sector, including the veterinary pharmaceutical industry. In Europe, the turnover for veterinary medicines is 5% of the turnover for medicines for human use – a veterinary product with a worldwide turnover of €10 million is a considered a relatively top-selling product.

The equivalent of orphan drugs in human medicines is available in veterinary medicinal products: minor use in minor species (MUMS, nowadays referred to as 'limited markets') is a growing problem. The limiting economic conditions make it not financially worthwhile to register products for rare indications in small populations. The human medicines industry only has to deal with one species – the veterinary industry needs to prove efficacy and safety in a multitude of species. Extrapolations from dog to cat, pig to chicken, or cow to sheep are not allowed. Within species from a legislative point of view there is even a difference between laying hens and broilers, piglets and sows and a non-ruminating calves and cows.

Veterinary medicines and food safety

Another important difference is that people are generally not eaten, whereas many animals are reared specifically for human consumption. This has consequences for the safe use of veterinary medicinal products. The awareness that residues of veterinary medicines in products of animal origin end up in food for human consumption was an important reason to mandate registration for veterinary medicinal products. Medicinal products for human consumption have had to be registered by the MEB since 1963, although requirements for veterinary medicines with regard to preparation, distribution and use were minimal. In 1986, the Veterinary Medicine Act was enacted. Based on this law, all veterinary medicines now have to be evaluated by the Dutch Ministry of Agriculture, Nature and Food Quality.

Synergy in the world of registration

In the past 20 years, much has changed in the world of registration. Legislation is made at a European level, and there is a great deal of   between the member states. As noted in earlier chapters, the CHMP has a veterinarian counterpart, the CVMP. And as mentioned elsewhere, there are committees for mutual and decentralised procedures for human and veterinarian use (the CMD(h) and the CMD(v)) that need to iron out differences in interpretation of the legislation.

Because the legislation is, for the most part, harmonised, registration procedures for human and veterinary medicines have a lot of similarities. This synergy has led to the transfer of the veterinary agency from the Ministry of Agriculture to the MEB.

The mandatory registration of veterinary medicinal products did, however, have consequences. In 1986, the first year of the legislation, between 1,000 and 2,000 applications were expected. In May 1987, around 5,500 applications had already been received. In 1988, a list of preliminary registries of medicinal products was published. Twenty years later, around 2,000 registered veterinary medicines are registered. The assumption that the number of registered veterinary medicines had decreased because many previously unregistered medicines were dangerous or ineffective, is incorrect. Most medicinal products disappeared because producers did not want to make the investments necessary to prove safety and efficacy according to the registration requirements. It can be concluded, however, that because of mandatory registration, the current registered veterinary medicinal products are safer than ever.

Rare diseases, orphan drugs and the MEB

by Bettie Voordouw

Rare diseases are those illnesses that occur so infrequently within any population that there is little or insufficient scientific and medical knowledge about them. The term 'orphan drugs' comes from the fact that medicinal products for rare diseases usually get little attention and are therefore neglected or 'orphaned'.

The definition of a 'rare disease' is not the same everywhere. In Europe, it means that the disease has to be severe and has been diagnosed in less than five in 10,000 people. In the US, this is seven in 10,000 people,[1] while an orphan disease in Australia can have only less than 2,000 occurrences, something that comes down to around one in 10,000, given that Australia has around 18 million inhabitants.

For the Netherlands, the European definition means that the disease cannot have been diagnosed in more than 8,000 patients. Worldwide, 6,000-7,000 rare diseases have been discovered and each week the medical professional literature describes around five new illnesses. An estimated 80% of these diseases are hereditary, which makes it an important problem.[2] Even though each individual rare disease accounts for only a small number of patients, the total number of patients suffering from a rare disease is estimated to be between 200,000 and 1,000,000,[1] and within the EU it would concern 30-35 million patients. Because most physicians will not come in contact with one of the few patients suffering one of the many possible rare diseases, as opposed to their contact with patients with, for example, type-2 diabetes, we cannot expect them to know all the specifics of the individual rare diseases. This often leads to long delays in diagnosing such illnesses, as well as leading to possible aggravation of the disease and, in those cases where a treatment is available, a delay of the start of the correct treatment.

Rare diseases are not just exotic. They include cystic fibrosis, Gaucher's disease, Familial Mediterranean Fever and some forms of cancer. They also include infectious diseases like malaria and tuberculosis.

Orphan drugs

Orphan drugs are medicinal products meant for the diagnosis, prevention or treatment of rare diseases. To obtain the status of 'orphan drug', the producer needs to prove that the product is indeed meant to treat a disease that falls under the category of rare diseases, and the potential that the medication has therapeutic value for the patient. A product can also obtain orphan drug status and the related financial and economic advantages if it is expected that, without such a designation, the drug will not become available to patients. The thinking behind this is that the expected financial gains do not justify possible costs and efforts to develop the medicine commercially. If a medicinal product is qualified as orphan, this does not automatically mean that the producer will never get any financial gain – on the contrary, sometimes large profits are made by the developer of an innovative orphan drug. A 2001 analysis showed that out of the ten best-selling biotech products in the US, five products initially qualified as orphan drugs. Importantly, aside from financial-economic interests, scientific interests primarily play a role in the decision to develop a medicinal product in the treatment of a rare disease.[3] For patients who suffer from a rare disease, it is important that the medicinal product they are treated with is as safe and efficacious as 'normal' medicinal products.

In fact, orphan drugs follow the same route when producers apply for an MA. The requirements of clinical studies for 'popular' medicinal products must also be met for smaller studies for orphan drugs. Although it was originally assumed that it would be difficult, if not impossible, to conduct research in orphan products that met all the standard requirements, most orphan drugs are based on controlled research, just like any other medicinal product. In a recent evaluation of 47 orphan drugs registered by the EMA using the centralised procedure until October 2007, more than 85% were based on Phase II research (in which the effect of a treatment is primarily researched using laboratory parameters) or Phase III research (indicating a better chance of survival, or a decrease in symptoms, than with other available treatments or no treatment at all). Around half of these studies were randomised and blinded.[4] It must be noted that research in orphan drugs treating rare oncology indications was based on Phase II research, whereas research for orphan drugs treating rare diseases in heart and pulmonary arteries is based on Phase III research. More than 50% of orphan drugs have been developed for treatment of oncology indications, followed by products for the treatment of musculoskeletal and nervous system diseases.

In order to conduct well-founded clinical studies with orphan drugs, international cooperation is essential to obtain a sufficient number of patients, and national patient organisations from different countries which joined forces have played an important role in this. For some diseases, even this effort is not enough. Very rare diseases distinguish themselves only by being recognised as an individual indication if the illness is very severe. Orphan drugs treating these patients, the so-called 'ultra orphans', can be registered using the description of individual patients. A special study in such a situation is the 'n=1-research', ie, research with a single patient. This makes it possible to have one patient participate in a study for an ultra orphan disease. Sometimes more than one medicinal product is compared successively in this one patient. Sometimes the treatment of diseases affecting the metabolism as a result of lack of enzymes (eg, Gaucher's disease) is relatively easy. An example occurs in patients whose concentration of ammonium in their blood is dangerously high because of a shortage of N-acetylglutamate-synthetase. This is an illness babies are born with, of which, in the Netherlands, less than five children suffer. The disease can be easily treated by administering carglumate acid. This compound lowers the ammonia levels in blood quickly, often within 24 hours. If treatment is started before permanent brain damage has occurred, normal growth and development of the baby seems possible. It is therefore important to administer this compound as early as possible, often directly after birth.

Another trait of orphan drugs is that they often concern very recent developments, eg, gene therapy. This means that they raise a lot of scientific interest but there are also many problems and hindrances to the marketing of the medicinal product. As an example, antisense therapy is a form of treatment for genetic disorders or infections. When the genetic sequence of a particular gene is known to be causative of a particular disease, it is possible to synthesise a strand of nucleic acid (DNA, RNA or a chemical analogue) that will bind to the messenger RNA (mRNA) produced by that gene and inactivate it, effectively turning that gene 'off'.

A specific problem is that many new developments have their origin in an academic and/ or scientific setting, in which the attention is focused on research and publication of such research. This attention is not necessarily in accordance with the requirements that need to be met in the registration procedure of an orphan drug, and the possible financing of the development of the regulatory course for the product. On the other hand, it is important that academic studies which have been conducted and financed for years should be able to contribute to the registration of a product. New developments of compounds or medicinal products that will reach the registration process will create a challenge for the developers of the product as well as for the competent authorities .

Committee for Orphan Medicinal Products (COMP)

Patients with a rare disease are as entitled to quality medical care as patients with more common illnesses. Because of this, policies have been developed over the past 20 years to stimulate the development of orphan drugs. The US enacted the Orphan Drug Act in 1983, and this was followed by the introduction of the European Directive on Orphan Drugs of 28 April 2000 (nr. 141/2000).

The EU included measures to promote the development of orphan drugs in the Directive; ten years of exclusive marketing rights and reduced tariffs. For the producer, the ten-year market exclusivity is the most important of these measures, as market exclusivity means that, for a period of ten years, the producer is the only company allowed to market that product for that registration. No similar product can be registered by the EMA or a member state for the same indication. In awarding orphan drug status, the pharmacological similarity (working mechanism, point of application) is the determining factor, whereas the CHMP defines 'similar' by looking at chemical-pharmaceutical similarities. A non-similar product can be registered for the same indication in the same period, and can obtain orphan drug status, with its own ten-year market exclusivity. This means that discussions on 'similarity' are very important, and will be for some time to come.

Only in very special circumstances can such ten-year market exclusivity be interrupted. Examples are the permission of the holder of the exclusivity, situations where the holder of that market exclusivity cannot produce enough of the medicinal product for patient requirements, or the competitor can prove that his product is superior to the original product. The Directive also gives the opportunity for member states to ask for a re-evaluation of the criteria five years after the orphan status has been obtained. Thus far this has not been done, but it may happen if there is doubt that the orphan drug criteria still apply. It is foreseen that as a therapy becomes available, the particular illness receives more attention, and more patients will be diagnosed, causing the disease to lose its 'rare' status.

The option of reducing tariffs is the most widely used of the available benefits for orphan drug development. If a medicinal product applies for an orphan drug MA, tariffs will be reduced by 50% and free scientific advice (protocol assistance) is available.

The Directive also forms the foundation for the COMP, one of the EMA committees. The COMP is responsible for the evaluation of applications for orphan drug status. It must determine if the indication that the medicinal product intends to diagnose, treat, or prevent is not prevalent in more than five in 10,000 inhabitants of the EU. Another option besides the prevalence criteria is the assumption that a disease might be not that rare but it is unlikely that the producer will see any return on its investment. This second criterion is rarely used. In the six years of the existence of the COMP, there have only been two cases of orphan drug status being awarded using this financial-economic criterion. Each application is also evaluated on a scientific basis; the questions to be answered are, first, if it is likely that the compound will be an effective medicinal product in the suggested indication, and second, if it will offer significant benefit to the patient.

The COMP's sole responsibility is its decision to award orphan drug status – the decision on marketing authorisation lies with the CHMP. The COMP does evaluate twice: once very early in the registration procedure, and once after the MA has been granted. The 'significant benefit' criterion plays an increasingly important role, primarily in the second evaluation. It should be established if there is another medicinal product available for the same indication, and if the new product is clearly something other than simply improved efficacy or composition, and it includes an evaluation of the product's contribution to a patient's care (eg, oral administration instead of intravenous administration). It is important that clinically relevant improvements can be proven when compared with a medicinal product that is already registered. Such evaluation is becoming more and more complex as more products become available, so producers are now advised of the use, and sometimes the necessity, of early scientific advice that they can get freely from the registration authorities.

The development of orphan drugs, significant benefit and the role of COMP

As noted, orphan drugs are entitled to free scientific advice, known as 'protocol assistance' by the Scientific Advice Working Party (SAWP). This advice relates to the development plan and the study plan, but also covers the requirements to determine significant benefit. This latter part of the advice is given by the COMP members in the SAWP – the significance of this aspect of scientific advice is often undervalued. The significant benefit criterion is very important because without it, the medicinal product will not continue to have orphan drug classification after the second evaluation, and so loses its exclusivity. It will remain registered, but without the privileges that the status of an orphan drug would bring.

This exclusivity appears the most complex part of the legislation around orphan drugs. The producer must prove that its product has significant benefit compared with medicinal products and treatments already on the market. All data that prove significant benefit must be in the dossier. In addition, non-pharmacological and therefore unregistered interventions, such as surgical treatments, diets or medical devices, can be considered acceptable treatments. Until December 2006, less than 50% of orphan drugs had applied for protocol assistance, and in two thirds of the applications, significant benefit was a topic of discussion.

Another issue is that an orphan drug indication is different from a therapeutic indication. A product can be registered for treatment of a kidney tumour after an earlier treatment has failed ('second line treatment') but the orphan drug indication is wider: 'treatment of kidney tumour'. With an increase in the number of products for the same orphan drug indications, significant benefit must play an ever more important role, and producers should make more use of protocol assistance.

Another responsibility of the COMP is to advise the European Commission on the development of policies for orphan drugs and to assist the Commission in creating Directives and international cooperation in the field of orphan drugs.

Orphan drugs and the role of the MEB

The MEB has represented the Netherlands in the COMP since May 2006. This makes sense, as applications are becoming more and more complex. The uncertainty for each medicinal product in development is great, and for orphan drugs this uncertainty is probably even greater. Though these uncertainties decrease during the course of a registration, strong support is very important.

The small number of patients, the development plans, the discussion around significant benefit and, above all, the novelty of a relatively great number of orphan drugs (and often small companies or academic centres who develop the same compounds), make the chances of tripping up somewhere along the registration path significantly more likely.

The WHO published a report, 'Priority Medicines for Europe and the World' in 2004, leading the Dutch government to start its own project of the same name, 'Priority Medicines'. This project aims to create an agenda for the development of medicinal products seen from a public healthcare point of view. As has been said before, the MEB is responsible for the evaluation and safeguarding of the efficacy, risks and quality of medicinal products. It does this by giving scientific advice, evaluation of applications for MAs and the promotion of safe and responsible use of medicinal products. The performance of this task is enabled by the strong position of the MEB in the Netherlands and in Europe.

References

[1] *www.weesgeneesmiddelen.nl*
[2] *S van Weely, C M A Rademaker, J S Huizer, H G M Leufkens. 'Zeldzame zorg binnen het takenpakket', Pharmaceutisch Weekblad, nr.11, 17 maart 2006.*
[3] *J Llinare-Garcia. 'Significant benefit assessment prior to marketing authorization', Presentation informal COMP, Lisbon October 2007.*
[4] *www.uvleuven.be/UZroot/content/Home/wieiswie/diensten/kindergeneeskunde/cardioloie/ziektebeelden/obb/*

18

Combination products – two worlds, one patient!

by Waldo Weijers

Border areas have always intrigued – places where the authorities and laws of one country necessarily give way, at the border crossing, to those of the neighbouring country. Sometimes these borders are a hotspot for conflicts, but they are also meeting points for people and cultures to trade and share knowledge. These meetings can sometimes lead to a new era, where one country's seemingly untouchable customs are replaced by the customs of its neighbour, and this despite language differences. Some pioneers in a strange land have even distinguished themselves by learning to speak the other country's language.

Medicines and medical devices are similar. They border each other, are related, and are sometimes required to cooperate with one another. A 'combination product' is a medical device with a supporting pharmaceutical compound. Medicinal products and medical devices differ from each other in terms of regulations, scientific research, production and last but not least, the people who work with them. In brief: they come from different worlds, but have a common goal – the health of that one patient.

History

Medicines have a much longer history of being regulated than medical devices. Some people may say, therefore, that medicines should have the rights of the eldest. Nationally, the oldest legislation written for medicines was the Dutch Medicines Act (WOG) of 1963, which was subsequently amended and extended via European legislation, and most recently revised in 2007.[1]

In all such legislation, one property in the definition of a medicine has remained constant: a medicine is still a product which is being used to cure or prevent a disease, defect, wound or pain, or to diagnose the same. In addition, products that restore, improve or change physiological functions can come under medicines legislation. All of these actions need to be achieved by using pharmacological, immunological or metabolic effects. The last part is crucial, especially in the eyes of professionals in the world of medicine.

The regulation of medical devices is much younger. The first Dutch national legislation dates from 1970, the first European Directives are from the 1990's,[2] while the most recent European legislation dates from September 2007[3] and this still has to be implemented in national legislation.

Applications for medicines and medical devices are similar in some ways. A medical device is a product which is used for diagnosing, preventing, guarding, treating or alleviating a disease, wound or handicap. Products used for research, replacement or change of the anatomy of a physiological process can also be medical devices. The same is true for products that control conception, like IUDs (intrauterine devices such as the spiral or the coil) or condoms. To be classified as a medical device, the efficacy should not be achieved by using pharmacological, metabolic or immunological means, which would make it a medicinal product. The working mechanism of a medical device has to be physical in nature, such as a mechanical action or a physical barrier (like condoms). The support of organs or bodily functions or the replacement thereof is included in the medical device category too.

Implementation of the European legislation for medical devices has caused a shift. Some products, previously considered medicines, suddenly became medical devices. A classic example is the IUD. The registration of this contraceptive device was cancelled when it came to be considered a medical device, and no longer a medicine. This certainly caused concern among some stakeholders in the strictly-regulated medical field, because IUDs were then no longer under the control of the medicines regulatory authorities and would be managed by the 'strangers' from the world of medical devices.

Differences between the two worlds

Medicines are regulated by the government officials and institutions that come under the responsibility of the government – in the Netherlands, the MEB. Elsewhere in Europe, the competent authorities evaluating MA applications are government institutions too. These competent authorities weigh the balance of the risks and benefits of new medicines and, when these prove positive, they grant an MA. These agencies do the evaluations themselves or bear the responsibility if they outsource them.

Medical devices are not evaluated by a governmental body, but by qualified organisations, the 'notified bodies'. In the Netherlands, the notified body is 'KEMA'. Notified bodies have received authorisation from their governments to evaluate medical devices and certify them. Following certification, the product receives the 'CE' mark.

Not every medical device needs to be approved by a notified body; this is only deemed necessary for the higher risk classified products, those that are classified as Class 2a/2b and 3. An example of a Class 1 product is a thermometer. For Class 1 devices, the manufacturer may assess if the product meets the specifications. An example of a Class 3 product is a cardiovascular stent. For Class 2 and 3 devices, the assessment is conducted by a notified body.

As the notified body is not a government body, it is not the competent authority for medical devices; in the Netherlands this is the IGZ. The IGZ also supervises the notified bodies. As the MEB is a government body, it is also the competent authority, therefore in the Netherlands there are two different competent authorities, one for medicines, the MEB, and one for medical devices, the IGZ.

The aforementioned differences between the two worlds relate to the differing regulations and assessment bodies. The real differences come to light when looking at the working methods and the way of thinking of the people who execute the rules. Some compare the assessment of medical devices with the certification process for an ISO certificate, which is a quality management system. At the time of approval of a device, not all details need to be finalised, though the essential requirements need to have been met. The working mechanisms need to be described clearly and the product must be clearly heading towards further improvement. Its progress is followed and, at previously determined moments, new evaluations are conducted and the approval is considered again. The above comparison to an ISO certification is correct and unsurprising. Evaluation for quality seals in general and for ISO in particular are the field of expertise of the notified bodies.

It is no secret that the different and stricter approach used for medicinal products is often considered, in the world of medical devices, to be too rigid and counter-productive to obtaining safe beneficial products that help the patient. In the medicinal world, however, it is thought that the method of temporary approval with a subsequent tract to improve is structured too loosely to be used responsibly with risk-carrying products (ie, medicines).

When worlds collide...

The combined evaluations relate to the consultation procedures for medical devices that contain a supporting pharmaceutical compound which, by itself, would come under the control of the medicines regulations. In this process, the notified bodies as well as the medicines regulatory authorities have a role. It can be said that, in Europe, the MEB is one of the more prominent players in these consultations and procedure evaluations. The MEB has cooperated with national and around ten foreign notified bodies in the evaluation process, with experience of around 60 consultation procedures. Some of these procedures are still ongoing.

The law states that the notified body is responsible for the entire evaluation of medical devices with a medicinal compound. The notified body is the one who grants a certification, not the medicines regulatory authority. The product is and will remain a medical device. Meanwhile, the notified body must seek advice from a medicines authority with regard to the medicinal compound – these are the aforementioned consultation procedures.

A consultation procedure often starts with a discussion about whether or not the consultation should be held. A demarcation document[4] can give guidance in this discussion, as this document defines the difference between a medical device and a medicine. It also gives examples of each category. It must be said, however, that some examples are based more on convention than clear logic. For example, while the previously mentioned IUD changed category from a medicine to a medical device, 'water for injections' is considered a medicine, [5] even though 'water' has a minor pharmacological profile. Combination products are even harder to qualify. The syringe is a medical device, the medication that is injected a medicine – that much is clear. A pre-filled syringe is categorised as medicine because 'if the device and the medicinal product form a single integral product which is intended exclusively for use in the given combination and which is not reusable, that single product is regulated as a medicinal product'. [6]

The consultation procedure concerns medical devices that do not originally contain a medicine, and as such are considered medical devices, but in which now, in support of their medical use, a pharmaceutical compound is integrated. An actual example is the drug-eluting stent. The stent was previously marketed as a bare stent, without the medicine. Recently, medicines aimed at slowing down cell growth in coronary arteries to avoid further clogging of the arteries were added. With these products, the notified body must seek advice from a medicines authority such as the MEB. In such cases the approach is very European; a German notified body can seek advice from the Dutch MEB. After the German notified body then certifies the product, it is admitted in all EU member states.

If the MEB acts as the medicines authority, it needs to give an evaluation of the pharmaceutical quality, safety and benefit of the added compound. The discussion is usually about the layout of the dossier as it is submitted by the producer of the medical device. Does this need to follow the strict rules of a dossier for a medicinal product or not? It now has become clear that a producer of medical devices cannot be expected to follow those strict guidelines, because its product is a medical device, for which less stringent rules are in place. However, evaluation of the supporting pharmaceutical compound needs to follow the rules for medicines. The form in which the information is presented might be different, but the content still needs to meet the criteria used to evaluate medicines. A following discussion could be on the extent to which the medicine authority can go, or must go, in its 'medicine-style' evaluation.

In the evaluation of medicines it is common practice, and endorsed in the guidelines, that a new medication is compared, during the research phase, with other medicines that are already accepted as 'gold standard' in the treatment of the illness. Comparison to an active comparator is not as common in the world of the medical devices. The possibility that there is another product available on the market with more added benefit need not be considered. The medicinal field argues that the utmost benefit for the patient always needs to be sought, which would include studies for the most beneficial product.

In recent times both worlds seem to have come together somewhat, possibly more because of safety issues than because of the benefit/efficacy discussion. There have been discussions, for example, about the long-term safety of drug-eluting stents. These discussions were not just about the character of the active compounds, but also the character of the polymer compounds used to bind the active compounds to the bare stent. Because of differences in both active and non-active compounds, depending on the type of stent and the producer, the idea that not all medical devices are the same has begun to get more support. So comparing a bearing product not just with a bare product but also with a similar bearing product is a small step.

Discussions as described above do have their value – they indicate that the players take each other seriously.

Where do we go from here?

A good roadmap for the future must be found in the increase of cooperation between the notified bodies and the competent authorities. This was first suggested by the GMT, the Directorate of Medicines and Medical Technology of the Dutch Ministry for Public Health, Welfare and Sport, and was considered a visionary approach.

As the Netherlands chaired the EU in 2004, the GMT invited the MEB to speak at the competent authority meeting for medical devices in Rotterdam, to sound out the views of the medical world. There was cause for concern as to how both worlds seemed to be too separate. To improve this, the MEB in cooperation with the GMT organised a symposium. Various assessors from the MEB gave presentations to experts from the notified bodies, who in turn were invited to give their views on cooperation, together with employees from the GMT and the IGZ. It transpired that the MEB saw the notified bodies as an applicant, just like an applicant for an MA. Meanwhile, the notified bodies considered themselves as the evaluating organisations, with a consulting role for the MEB.

Enlightened by the differing views expressed and subsequently discussed at this symposium, the MEB has since found other ways to communicate with employees from the notified bodies, such as the possibility for scientific advice as well as pre-submission meetings, similar to the meetings held for MAs. The MEB also supplies safety information to the notified bodies, which will be mandatory following the latest Directive.[7]

There are enough positive starting points for improvements. Notified bodies are showing increasing interest in the intensive system of pharmacovigilance that is used for medicines. At the same time, in the field of medicines evaluation, there is some discussion about a risk-oriented approach to such evaluations. The focus is already there on the critical parts of the process. Added to this, conditional approvals are not unheard of nowadays in the medicinal world.

It seems that the worlds are coming together a little. A next step could be that reviewers from the notified bodies and evaluators from the medicines authorities work together on one product. There may well come a point where the MEB and the notified bodies participate together in a meeting to discuss the aspects of each other's evaluations, and present those to the college of the MEB.

Looking back at the introduction to this article about borderlines as a place where people share knowledge and learn from each other, there is an important challenge for all involved. Two different worlds or not, it is the wellbeing of the individual patient that counts.

References

[1] Directives 65/65/EEC, 75/318/EEC, 75/319/EEC, 75/319/EEC, 2001/83/EU, 2004/27/EU{o}.

[2] Directives 90/385/EEC, 93/42/EEC and 98/79/EU.

[3] Directive 2007/47/EU.

[4] Guidance document MEDDEV 2.1/3 rev 2, July 2001 'Demarcation between: Directive 90/385/EEC on Active Implantable Devices. Directive 93/42/EEC on Medical Devices and Directive 65/65/EEC relating to Medicinal Products and related Directives', European Commission DG Enterprise Directorate G, Unit 4.

[5] Article A 4.2 Guidance document MEDDEV 2.1/3 rev 2, July 2001.

[6] Article A 6.2 Guidance document MEDDEV 2.1/3 rev 2, July 2001.

[7] Preamble Directive 2007/47 EC.

19

Appealing MEB decisions

by Melita van der Mersch

This chapter describes the legal protection for industry against decisions made by the MEB and, according to the numerous complaints, there is a lot that needs to be improved. These complaints are primarily from legal experts assisting the industry, and they cover two different aspects:

- Decisions by the MEB are only marginally tested by the national court system
- A complaint about a decision in a mutual recognition procedure that holds judicial or factual errors needs to be filed in all European member states.

If these complaints are true, are improvements necessary?

Appeals in the Netherlands

A decision to grant, deny, or change an application can be appealed as well as a decision to change the delivery status.. Only individuals and companies directly involved – the interested parties – can challenge a decision. The applicant is an interested party; his competitors can be interested parties. The holder of a licence for a reference medicine is considered to have a third-party interest and thus can also appeal MEB decisions.

In the appeals procedure, the MEB reconsiders its earlier decision on the advice of the appeal commission. The appeal commission consists of the head of the MEB, one of the other MEB members, the lawyer/adjunct-secretary and an MEB secretary. All documents available at the time of the appeal need to be considered, as well as new (research) data if these become available during the appeal. If the new data lead to a different decision, the appeal is granted. This decision can be appealed again by an interested party. The procedure is in front of a civilian court, and the judge will consider if the MEB was reasonable in its initial decision. Even if the civil court assumes the MEB has sufficient expertise to come to the correct decision, this could be disputed if the interested parties can prove that a particular expertise was not available to the MEB.

The possibilities to challenge the contents of an MEB decision are limited, for obvious reasons. Any application for an MA undergoes an extensive evaluation which has its own safeguards. However, the law does offer possibilities to challenge the content of an MEB decision. In such cases, the parties must have an expert who can challenge the content of the decision.

To increase efficiency in the decision-making process, it is recommended that complaints of interested third parties are already voiced during the evaluation of the application by the MEB. The applicant has many possibilities to voice reservations about the preliminary decisions – an interested third party with complaints currently does not have a similar opportunity during the application assessment procedure. However, the law does entitle an interested third party to issue such a complaint. The MEB needs to hear an interested third party before a decision on the application is made. Article 4:8 Awb states that:

1. Before making an administrative decision about which an interested party who has not applied for the administrative decision may be expected to have reservations, an administrative authority shall give that interested party the opportunity to state his views, if:

   (a) the administrative decision is based on information about facts and interests relating to the interested party, and

   (b) this information was not supplied in the matter by the interested party himself.

2. Subsection 1 shall not apply if the interested party has not complied with a statutory obligation to supply information.

This may occur in an application for an MA for a generic medicinal product. The MAH for the reference product is likely to have complaints regarding the issuing of an MA. By hearing this third party, the MEB can evaluate possible objections and decide on them in advance. This can avoid appeals of decisions. During the evaluation phase, all data are usually confidential; this also applies for interested third parties, so the MEB can only offer comments on the procedure after the application is concluded. This can be done in the public evaluation report, which is published by the MEB after the decision on the application is taken.

Appealing decisions in Europe

If an applicant for an MA wants to register in more than one EU member state, he or she must follow one of the two possible procedures mentioned in earlier chapters – the MRP and the DP.

If member states disagree with each other or with the applicant during either procedure, the issue can be raised with the CHMP. The committee issues well-founded advice to the European Commission, which will in turn issue a draft decision according that advice. All parties involved now have a chance to give their comments and, following this, the European Commission will issue a binding decision. This decision can deny the MA. In such cases an appeal is possible through the European Court of Justice. This procedure is between the applicant and the member states – there is no role for third parties. The only possible way an MAH of a reference product can take is that of the appeal in each individual member state against the issuance of an MA of a generic product. As each country has a different legal system this is often very complicated, costly and time-consuming.

Member states can of course avoid procedures by independently cancelling or suspending the MA if the judge in another member state decides to do so. There have been many appeals against decisions in MRPs; thus far, none of the disputed MAs has been cancelled.

Conclusion

Opportunities for interested third parties to appeal decisions need to be improved, particularly in European procedures; an interested third party does not have the opportunity to have his opinions on the decision process heard. Neither do they have appeal possibilities if they disagree with a decision. The authorities too will benefit from interested third party input, and the regulation thereof in European legislation. Processing many informal letters and requests takes time, time that could be saved if there were a fixed moment when interested third parties could have the chance to give input. An authority holds a stronger position in an appeal if it can prove that all grievances were already considered during the application procedure, and national procedures can be avoided.

Medicines without borders – ICH and FDA

by Jan Willem van der Laan

Medicines do not have geographical borders. Multinational pharmaceutical companies have MAs in many European member states, but the development of most of their medicinal products takes place elsewhere in the world. What follows are some examples of international cooperation by the MEB.

Benelux

Cooperation in Europe started on a small scale, in the Benelux committee in the early 1980s. Luxembourg is a small country and therefore some of the members from the Luxembourg committee were from the Netherlands and some were from Belgium. The atmosphere was friendly but not completely trusting. If Belgium or Luxembourg was assigned to be the leader on a project, the Netherlands conducted a shadow assessment according to MEB regulations. Trust is something that needs to grow. When the Benelux committee was disbanded after a short time, continued cooperation with Belgium was encouraged by nominating a Belgian pharmacy professor as a member of the MEB.

Europe

There has been European cooperation for some time in study groups and guidelines. The first Directive, 65/65, dates from 1965. Directives 75/318 and 75/319 were issued in the 1970s. These last two give the regulations for medicinal products, which are still to some extent part of the newer Directive 2001/83, in which the Directives from 1965 through 2001 are combined. Regulations are binding and Directives are adapted into law and as such are mandatory for companies. Guidelines, on the other hand, give recommendations that companies can follow, but that they also can divert from, as long as they give their justification for doing so. Factual cooperation started primarily in the sphere of writing of the guidelines. This was done in working parties (discussed in Chapter 8) in which experts from each member state have a seat. The permanent Working Parties of the CHMP are:

- Biologics Working Party (BWP)
- Efficacy Working Party (EWP)
- Joint CHMP/CVMP Quality Working Party (QWP)
- Pharmacovigilance Working Party (PhVWP)
- Safety Working Party (SWP)

Other working parties mentioned in Chapter 8 consist of special experts rather than members representing their countries.

Creating guidelines

Some guidelines are created after years of discussions and exchange of arguments. For example, in the early 1980s, attempts were made to coordinate the labelling of medicinal products for use during pregnancy (the so-called 'categorisation' used in Australia and adopted in Sweden, which at that time was not a member of the EU) within Europe. These attempts were unsuccessful, primarily because of opposition from France. The guideline was then was shelved for many years. It was not until 2001 that new efforts were made to coordinate labelling, as people slowly began to realise that the safety of medicinal products during pregnancy could not be described in the suggested five categories. The fact that it took seven years after the restart to come to a finished document shows that it was a complex issue.

ICH

The ICH process started in Europe. The full name of the ICH is the International Conference on Harmonisation on Technical Requirements for Pharmaceuticals for Human Use. It is a partnership of six parties, called the 'six-pack' (see Table 2).

When cooperation within the CPMP really began in the late 1980s, the head of the Unit Pharmaceuticals of the Directorate-General Enterprise, at that time the DGIII, in Brussels, took the initiative to widen international harmonisation. This led to the first ICH meeting in 1991 – indeed a visionary action (see Table 3).

Regulatory Parties	Industrial Parties
1 European Union (including CHMP)	4 European Federation of Pharmaceutical Industry Associations (EFPIA)
2 US Food and Drug Administration	5 Pharmaceutical Research Manufacturers Association (PhRMA)
3 Japanese Ministry of Health Labor & Welfare (now including PMDA)	6 Japanese Pharmaceutical Manufacturers Association (JPMA)
Secretariat: International Federation of Pharmaceutical Manufacturers & Associations	

Table 2: '*Six-pack*' *– International Conference on Harmonisation.*

The central coordination is in the hands of the International Federation of Pharmaceutical Research Associations (IFPMA) in Geneva (see www.ICH.org). The WHO has been an observer in this process from the beginning, but there is a long list of observers; Health Canada, the European Free Trade Association (primarily Switzerland, also including Norway and Iceland), Australia, and China and from the industry's side; the International Generics Program to represent producers of generic medicinal products, and the Biologics Industries Organization (BIO).

The highest authority within the ICH is the Steering Committee (SC), in which only representatives of the 'six-pack' formally have a seat and voting rights. The SC decides the process and the initiatives, and has to approve the final guidelines.

It is a misunderstanding to see the ICH as an institution that independently issues guidelines. The real harmonisation role is played by the Expert Working Groups (EWGs) to which all parties can nominate one or two members and perhaps one or more experts, which happens quite regularly.

In the early days, there was hardly any experience with this type of work, and the procedures were not described in detail. There was no strong drive to the process, and there was a lot of work to be done. In 1991 there were three quality subjects, four safety subjects and four efficacy subjects. At that time, the SCs and the EWGs met three times a year in one of the regions. To announce the results of these discussions to the public, two large annual conferences were organised, although this later changed to one conference every three years. When most guidelines were created, the frequency of the meetings held by the SC and the EWG meetings changed to twice a year, and currently there are no more general conferences (see Table 3).

ICH	Year	Place
ICH 1	1991	Brussels
ICH 2	1993	Orlando
ICH 3	1995	Yokohama
ICH 4	1997	Brussels
ICH 5	2000	San Diego
ICH 6	2003	Osaka

Table 3: *Frequency and location of Steering Committee and Expert Working Group meetings between 1991 and 2003.*

The impact of the guidelines is enormous. In the clinical field, the 'Guideline on Good Clinical Practice' (E6) is the most important; it has achieved legal status in the Netherlands.

The procedure

The procedure (see Figure 4) is as follows:

A topic can be put on the agenda if all parties agree, and a Concept Paper, which also gives a timeframe, is written (Step 1). Next, the EWG begins writing a first draft. All six parties need to be in agreement, and they sign for this in a Step 2 document. The various authorities take the document and publish it through their usual means. The EMA has its own website and the FDA has its Federal Register. The latter is often a time-consuming and therefore delaying process. In Step 3 the opportunity is given, for three to six months, to comment through the authorities. After this time the EWG meets again to determine the definitive text, Step 4. All six parties are part of this final round. Next the regulators sign the documents, and the documents finally need to be confirmed by the authorities and be given legal status. From this it is clear that the ICH itself is not able to give legal status to a document.

EU/EMA and FDA in ICH

The European delegation in the ICH is led by a delegation of the EU, not by the EMA. This indicates that the EMA does not have the same status as its American counterpart, the FDA. The FDA delegation consists of evaluators, and sometimes researchers, from the FDA, whereas the experts from the EU delegation are from the authorities of the member states.

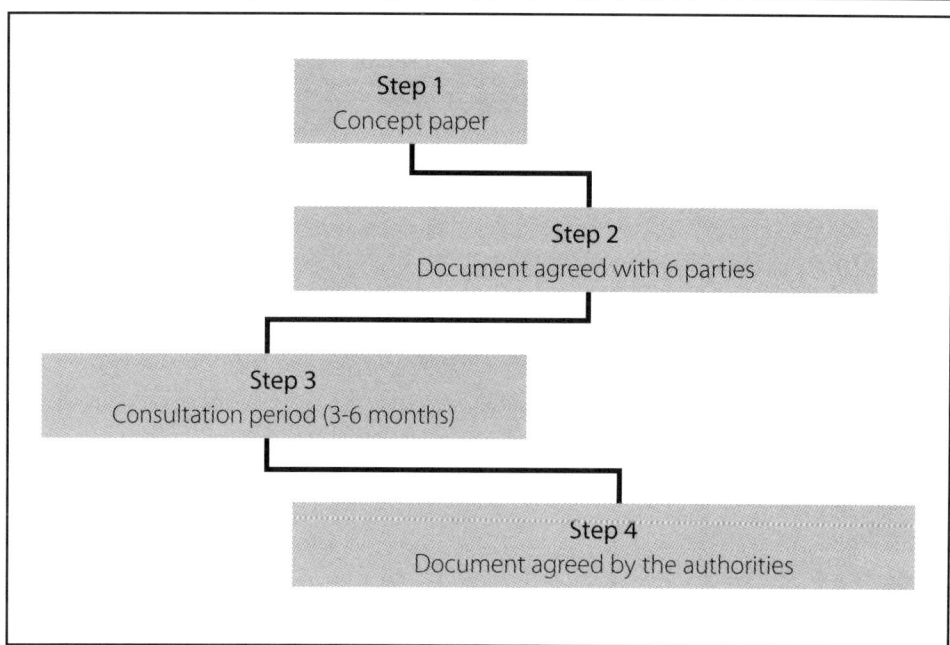

Figure 4: *The 'six-pack' procedure.*

This difference is sometimes hard to explain to outsiders. In recent years, EMA employees have become more knowledgeable and, in general, they maintain the idea that the EMA's status is the same as that of the FDA.

ICH results

International coordination is very important, and the first results are also often the best. This is best demonstrated by giving examples from the nonclinical safety field, the field of animal experimental pharmacology and toxicology. There were some early successes during the first ICH in Brussels in 1991, three of which were:

- *Harmonisation of acute toxicity.* Public pressure to take better care of laboratory animals led to a discussion on the necessity of the so-called LD50-test, a test from which many animals die. It soon became clear that an agreement could be reached by emphasising the no observable effect level (NOEL) dose, and particularly the no observable adverse effect level (NOAEL) dose.

- *Translations.* Language barriers cause trouble for the authorities. As an example, one Japanese term for NOAEL was translated incorrectly from Japanese into English, giving the wrong impression to Western toxicologists. 'Mu Sayo Ryo' stands for no-effect-dose and 'Mu Dokusei Ryo' stands for no-toxic-effect-dose. The difference between those two is the incorrect interpretation of the effect as 'toxic' as 'adverse'. In an attempt to avoid confusion, the Japanese added a third term, 'Mu Eikyo Ryo', meaning a dose without any biological effect, which in fact was the same as one of the earlier terms, thus causing even more confusion. Harmonisation at this point was primarily a case of correct translation (Hayashi, 1991).

- *Reproductive toxicity.* In Japan, the primary evaluation was done on an administrative level without specific toxicological knowledge. The exposure of rats and rabbits during pregnancy will be during a standard period, eg, from day 5 to day 16, but this can differ for various authorities, eg, from day 6 to day 18. As Japan was especially strict in applying this rule, studies sometimes had to be repeated because the Japanese requirements were not met. It has now been agreed that small differences in intervals will not lead to a new study.

Following the quick successes during the first ICH meeting in Brussels, many more topics have been discussed. As of 2006, ten quality guidelines, eight safety guidelines, fourteen efficacy guidelines and five multidisciplinary guidelines have been issued, some of them divided into A and B, and even C guidelines.

Common Technical Document (CTD)

Something we, as assessors, deal with every day is the development of a CTD, a joint index of a dossier for medicinal products. This was of primary interest to the industry parties, who put considerable time and effort into it. The registration authorities stayed on the sideline on this subject, realising the costs it would take and the fact that it was not to their immediate benefit. It is important to note that the CTD is only a standard index of a dossier. Whether or not a study should be conducted is regulated in a guideline, eg, for immunotoxicology, ICH S8. Once this study is done, the CTD will indicate where in the dossier the study should be placed, ie, Module 4.7.2.

Combining of dossier requirements thus far had only led to an enumeration of requirements. Europe wanted an expert report, a critical overview of the data in which the producer took responsibility for the choices he or she made when developing the product, including a table of all the studies. The FDA wanted a summary of every study, without the producer's opinion. The European philosophy is that the producer is responsible for its product and its defence thereof. The American philosophy is that the evaluator must be able to form his own opinion, without any influence from the producer.

The nonclinical part of the CTD now asks for an overview, the old expert report and the summaries. This works very well. When creating an evaluation report, the usually shorter review can be used as a basis, and the summaries can be used for filling in the gaps. It is always surprising that such interesting discussions about evaluation philosophies can be held about something as boring as an index of an evaluation dossier.

ICH culture

Each representative brings his or her own culture to the table. Americans are very direct, Japanese are very reticent. These of course are generalisations, and there are many exceptions. However, if a Japanese person says 'yes' this means, the first time, that they have understood the question, not that they agree – a very important aspect in the negotiations.

The ICH culture is also created by the 'caucus deliberations'. Each partner has their own meeting from 5.30pm until 7.00pm, during which the day's business is reviewed. Each EWG is discussed, and sometimes a strategy is determined. Europe also has a combined meeting of industry and regulators, which is chaired in turn by the members of the ICH steering committee of either of them. It is important to estimate correctly when it is your turn as an expert, because it is often hard to follow the other party's topics.

It is believed that the other parties all meet separately. The openness that the EU has towards industry seems to apply less in the US. Part of the culture is the way of life in the US where, among others, the government is highly concerned about legal claims which might result in vast damages payments. For this reason, all documents need to be checked by lawyers on all legal aspects before finalisation. If this can be done quickly during the meeting, this is not a problem. It is harder if this has to be done at a later date, and if previously agreed wording needs to be changed.

The legal tournament – an anecdote

There was a time when the Safety EWG was working on a revision of the documents from the first round, and found that, for one document (S1C for insiders), a problem was easily resolved by omitting a single word. All parties were happy with this solution and it was accepted. There were a few more changes, but these were quickly dealt with. Then the FDA lawyer took his turn at reading the document and had a few second thoughts about a part of the text that had not been changed, and was in fact established ten years previously. Now, the word 'acceptable' was no longer acceptable, and needed to be changed to 'appropriate'. The Japanese expert stated however that at some points in the text, the word 'acceptable' was more appropriate than the word 'appropriate', and so he deemed the substitution 'unacceptable'. Considerable time then had to be spent to find wording that was 'appropriate' as well as 'acceptable'.

We can learn from this story that America's legal culture is a part of the business that we have to accept, and that thought tipped the scales in coming to a conclusion together. You cannot harmonise everything. You have to bear in mind that you are dealing with regulations for medicinal products, but you cannot harmonise all the medical practices. That is true for Europe, but even more so for the entire world.

The US Food and Drug Administration

The US FDA is the main counterpart to the EU's EMA within the ICH. It is therefore important to mention some specifics about that agency here. The FDA is a very large organisation that holds many of the functions of a medicinal authority. In the Netherlands, and also in some other European countries, many of these activities are more spread out among various institutions that are independent from each other. (For the structure of the FDA, see the agency's website at www.fda.gov).

The FDA consists of centres that each have their own field of expertise. There is a centre for food, a centre for medical devices, a centre for drug evaluation and research (the CDER) and a centre for biologics evaluation and research (the CBER). The CDER is divided into 15 divisions, each of them covering different therapeutic fields.

Working with medicines, we mostly deal with the CDER and CBER. The different fields of these two centres are roughly the same as in the Netherlands own BMT (centrum voor

Biologische Geneesmiddelen en Medische Technologie) and KCF (Centrum voor Kwaliteit van Chemisch-Farmaceutische producten), both part of the RIVM. In Germany, the division would be between BfArM (Bundesinstitut für Arzneimittel und Medicinal Produkte) and PEI (Paul-Ehrlich-Institut).

Recently, the FDA has moved the evaluation of recombinant proteins from the CBER to the CDER, leading to many discussions about application of the guidelines for biological medicinal products and thus the recombinant proteins.

In general, the CBER has been more flexible in applying the rules than the CDER. This centre's stricter interpretation of the guidelines is the cause of great frustration within the pharmaceutical industry, and is one reason to start a new ICH process about safety measures for biological medicines.

Temporary FDA employee

As EU Topic Leader on Carcinogenicity I participated in the Expert Working Group on this topic. After finalising the first guideline (S1A on the need for carcinogenicity studies) in which we discussed the perspective for the next decade and the use of transgenic models (just starting to be evaluated), the FDA expert proposed that the next Guideline (S1B, choice of species) to include these transgenic models as a second choice, even without evaluation. Because of this difference in insight, the FDA representative invited me to become a temporary FDA employee for a month. As a result of this, we had a much better understanding of the regulatory atmosphere in EU and US systems in the nonclinical field.

Conclusion

The registration of medicinal products in the Netherlands has been controlled for many years by European procedures, and has long lost its solely national character. It is a fact of life that we are European citizens. Being a world citizen is an experience that is felt particularly in the ICH. As being involved in a multicultural environment leads to many stimulating (and sometimes frustrating) experiences, it is a challenge to be able to work in such an atmosphere.

Bibliography

Y Hayashi. 'The current situation with regard to No Effect Dose vs No Toxic Effect Dose', in P F D'Arcy and D W G Harron (Eds.), Proceedings of the First International Conference on Harmonisation, Brussels; 1991.

21 *Mind the gap!*

by Josee Hansen

Without safe medicinal products there is no safe care, but a safe medicine only leads to safe patient care if it is prescribed properly, delivered safely and properly used. There is a gap between the levels of precautionary and safety measures regarding the medicinal products before entering the market and the healthcare environment in which the medicinal product is indicated, prescribed, delivered and used. Figure 5 illustrates this discrepancy.

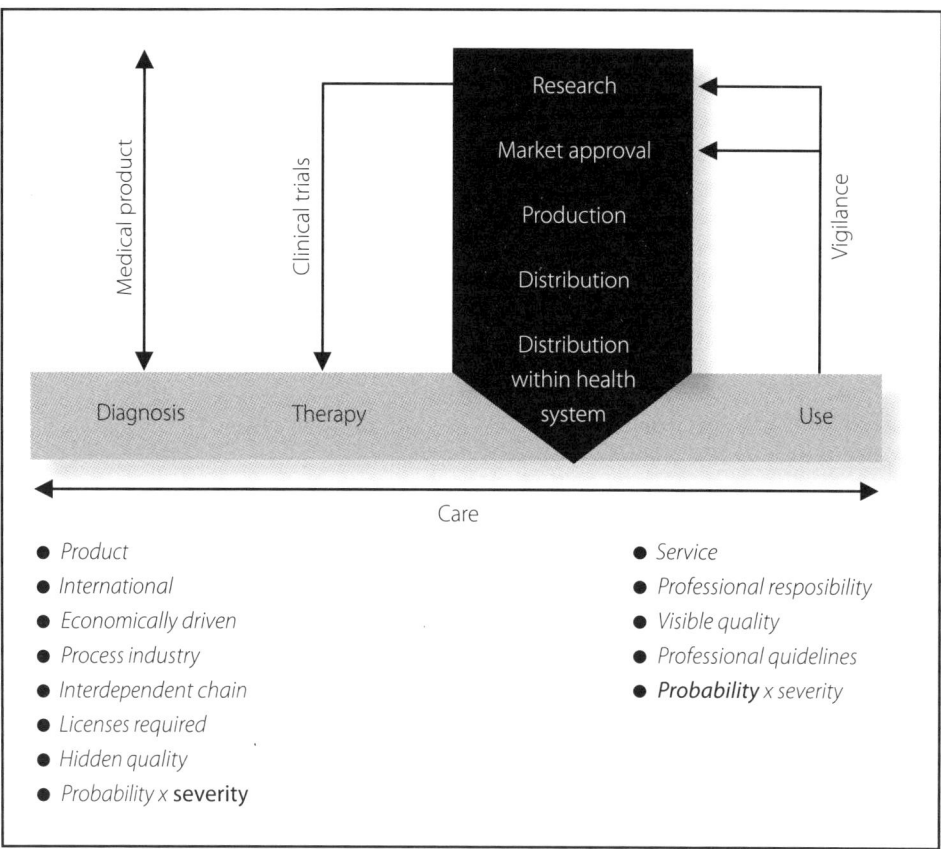

Figure 5: *Product cycle and care cycle for medicinal products.*

The regulatory approach to contain the risk of the medicinal product differs essentially from healthcare regulation. The Medicines Act and its annexes describe a set of detailed requirements, which are assessed and inspected before a medicinal product enters the market. The Quality of Healthcare Institutions Act (KZ), which regulates quality in healthcare, describes quality requirements for healthcare in global terms. A healthcare professional is allowed to deliver healthcare and is allowed clinical freedom to a large extent.

The two systems meet at the point where the medicinal product is dispensed, in the pharmacy. The pharmacist delivers medication – which is the medicinal product individualised to a specific patient – to the patient according to the physician's prescription. The considerations of the physician to prescribe are often unknown, and may differ to a great extent from the indications according to the carefully considered indications, dosages, etc, specified in the SmPC. The high rate of off-label prescribing reflects this.

Following this, the patient receives the medicinal product and starts using it. The non-compliance, non-concordance, incorrect use, or non-use of prescribed medicinal products is common for some medications, which obviously influences the success of the therapy.

Every patient must be able to rely on the fact that the medicinal product he or she is using has a positive risk–benefit ratio. As can be seen from previous chapters, the MEB has assessed this balance. The Inspectorate will have inspected the product's manufacture, in compliance with Good Manufacturing Practice; the distribution of the medicinal product is in compliance with Good Distribution Practice; and pharmacovigilance by the manufacturer aims to ensure the evaluation of adverse events in the use of the medicinal product.

The KZ requires that a healthcare provider should provide responsible care. This care needs to be effective, suitable, geared towards the patient, and of proven good quality. Stakeholders in the field, including healthcare workers, patients and insurance companies, need to further fulfil these requirements. There are no strict rules or regulations applied at the outset in this arena, as there are with medicinal products, but instead rules and regulations are determined by stakeholders and professional organisations.

The unauthorised or incorrect use of a medicinal product occurs quite often in the field of healthcare. One example is that of a medication being prescribed for a different indication than has been approved by the regulators – the so-called 'off-label' prescription, which is usually well-intentioned by the prescribing physician. Other examples include where the PIL is not read or not properly understood, or where the patient does not take the medicine according to the prescriber's instructions.

In brief, the assurance of the quality and safety of a licensed medicinal product is many times better than the assurance of correct prescribing and use. To establish if a medicine is prescribed and dispensed to meet the requirement of responsible care is not easy. In order to be able to provide data on this issue, the IGZ together with stakeholders and healthcare professionals has developed performance indicators. The gap, however, between the safeguards of a medicinal product assured at registration and its everyday use continue to exist.

The question, of course, is how can we bridge this gap? Built-in safety of any medicinal product is needed – everyone agrees on that. Not just because without it, safe care is not possible, but also because the impact of an unsafe medicinal product is enormous. It affects a large number of patients and the effects can spread out over a long period of time. So safety first is the rule. But how do we promote correct use? This is something we need to look into further. The cooperation between all competent authorities involved contributes to an increase in the safe use of medicinal products, and to a decrease in the quality gap.

22 *The MEB and the RIVM are inseparable*

by Hans Ovelgönne

The National Institute for Public Health and the Environment (RIVM) has been involved with the work of the MEB for a long time. It performs parts of the scientific evaluation of the registration applications on behalf of the MEB, in the field of safety and quality. The RIVM has more than 50 employees, primarily working in two centres – the State Laboratory for Biological Medicines (BMT) and the Centre for Quality of Chemical-Pharmaceutical Products (KCF). There are three fields in which the RIVM works for the MEB:

- The preclinical section of the registration dossier. This section contains all data of a medicinal product that are collected using animal experiments. This is evaluated by employees of the Pharmacological-Toxicological Evaluations (FTB).
- The quality section of the registration dossier as far as it concerns biotechnological medicines. This section describes the production methods of biotechnological medicines, and also touches on viral safety. This is evaluated by the employees of the Bio-Technological Medicinal Products (BTG).
- The quality section of the registration dossier as far as it concerns synthetic medicinal products. This section describes the production methods of medicines produced with chemical methods, and is evaluated by employees of the KCF.

Each of these groups has its own, sometimes long, history. This chapter describes how they got together in their current form at the RIVM.

FTB or 'the RIVM'

The preclinical evaluators assess the safety of new medicinal products by using laboratory and animal studies in the process of an MA evaluation. Of all evaluation groups within the RIVM, the FTB has the longest common history with the MEB as well as with the RIVM; this is noticeable if the MEB Board members ask the RIVM delegates questions, tending to address just the FTB.

The RIVM has been involved with preclinical assessments since the inception of the MEB in 1963. The two Board members responsible for preclinical evaluations both worked for the RIV, the predecessor of the RIVM.

Initially, Board members themselves wrote the evaluation reports on which the Board based its decisions. This later changed as the reports were written by RIV employees other than members of the MEB Board. The responsibility for compiling preclinical reports remained with the RIV, more specifically their Laboratory for Pharmacology.

At this time, the quality of the medicinal product was evaluated by the RIGO, in Leiden. Biological products such as vaccines and blood products were not yet regulated by the medicines legislation, but were evaluated by the National Control Laboratory (RCL), at RIV.

In 1984, the RIV merged with the National Institute for Drinking Water Supply and the Institute for Waste Research, to form the current RIVM. The Laboratory for Pharmacology merged with the RCL to create the Laboratory for Medicines and Medical Devices, LGM, the current BMT. Within the BMT, the FTB, a group of about eight evaluators, is responsible for preclinical evaluations.

BTG: the quality of biotechnological medicines

The BTG is, with the FTB, part of the BMT centre. This group has its origins in the former RCL of the RIVM, and was already, before the merger, occasionally involved in the evaluation of recombinant DNA medicinal products. These were registered since the 1980s in Brussels, in the so-called Concertation Procedure, the predecessor of the Centralised Procedure of the EMA. BTG currently evaluates the pharmaceutical quality of medicinal products of bio(techno)logical origin. This group of products includes vaccines, blood products and medicines produced using recombinant DNA techniques. They differ from chemical medicines because they cannot always be completely analysed. They are often complex protein mixtures. To safeguard the quality of these products, the BTG evaluates the production process carefully. If the quality of the final product cannot be fully guaranteed by data analysis, the producer needs to prove that the production process was controlled in such a way that the final product is of consistent quality. Changes in the production process are not readily accepted.

BTG has its roots in the registration of blood products and vaccines. Admission of these products to the market was traditionally regulated differently from other medicinal products. On the one hand, vaccines and blood products were initially not considered as medicines, while on the other hand, these products carry different risks, as blood products can carry illnesses. These products are still under a strict regimen. They have to be approved by the MEB and each produced batch has to be evaluated by a governmental laboratory. This evaluation consists of extensive safety tests, and an evaluation of the documentation of the producer. Before 1993, the admission of blood products and vaccines was determined by two acts: the Act on Sera and Vaccinations and the Act on Human Blood.

The Act on Sera and Vaccinations

The former Act on Sera and Vaccinations created a commission, Commission ex. Article 14. This commission was the responsibility of the Dutch Health Council (Gezondheidsraad), an independent advisory board charged with providing the government with scientific advice on public health Issues.[1] The members of commission ex. Article 14 were nominated to this function because of their position in healthcare organisations. Members were the lead inspector for medicinal products, the head of National Control Laboratory (RCL; the National Controller) and the Director-General of the RIVM – the latter was the head of the commission. The commission was responsible for the admission, the release, the clinical studies, and inspections of all vaccines and sera. The scientific evaluation was the responsibility of the RCL, as were the evaluation of the dossier and release of the batches of the product. The Director-General of the RIVM, as head of the commission ex. Article 14, decided on the release of batches of RIVM-vaccine, where he was also responsible for the production. In the late 1980s the notion grew that the RIVM as producer needed to meet the same requirements as other producers of vaccines, especially the independent evaluation. As of that moment, the RIVM began submitting their own dossiers. At this time the development of monoclonal antibodies began. These are antibodies that are produced in laboratories and do not contain a human or animal blood compound. These monoclonal antibodies are considered sera and therefore do not fall under the general Dutch Medicines Act, but under the Act on Sera and Vaccinations. They are evaluated by the commission in cooperation with the MEB because the products require European registration, the then-called Concertation Procedure of the CPMP, predecessor of the CHMP.

The Act on Human Blood

The Act on Human Blood created the Commission ex. Article 1. This commission advised the minister about the admission of blood products that could be kept for an extended period of time, ie, medicinal products made with blood plasma. The Commission ex. Article 1 also had members that were nominated because of their function in other organisations. The head of this commission was also the Director-General of the RIVM; the secretary was the National Controller. Release by batch was only mandatory for imported products, and no laboratory research was necessary. Products produced by the Central Laboratory for Blood transfusion services (CLB; the current Sanquin) were not released by the government in those days. During the 1980s, the CLB was considered a producer too, and finally they too had to submit a dossier with Commission ex. Article 1.

In 1993, two European Directives from the European Commission were implemented in the Dutch legislation, which changed the situation drastically for vaccines and blood products – from this time on, these products would be categorised under medicinal products.[2]

Because of this change, the Act on Sera and Vaccines and the Act on Human Blood were repealed, and the Dutch Medicines Act was amended. Vaccines and blood products now are considered medicinal products and are evaluated by the MEB. Some of the members of the aforementioned organisations became members of the MEB. For the compilation of evaluation reports, the existing expertise of the BTG was used. This change happened in a period of social concern about blood products because of the emergence of the HIV virus. In the Netherlands too, patients received contaminated blood, contracted the virus and died. Concerns about the transfer of Hepatitis C were in the media too, creating another headache for the MEB. The BTG has made great efforts to obtain the virological expertise to evaluate the safety of these products. This is also a difficult problem because of the shortage of blood products. If the safety requirements become too strict, and too many donations are rejected, haemophilia patients will undoubtedly suffer.

The practice of release per batch was still used within the existing infrastructure of the BTG. This was legally determined for blood in the Dutch Decision for Blood Products, and for vaccines in the Dutch Decision on Immunological Pharmaceutical Products. The competent authority was originally planned to be the IGZ; this authority now has been transferred to the RIVM.

In 1994, the BTG became the sole organisation to evaluate medicinal products made using the recombinant DNA technology. Prior to this, the RIGO, now KCF, evaluated these proteins, sometimes seeking biotechnological advice from the BTG. These products, eg, insulin, which were originally derived from animal sources, had been classified as medicinal products early on.

With the latest reorganisation, the shift in categorisation of medicinal products, blood products and vaccines to a categorisation of medicinal products of chemical origin and medicinal products of biological origin was complete. The current BTG group has ten evaluators.

KCF: The quality of chemical medicinal products

The KCF evaluates the quality of medicinal products for human use as well as for veterinarian use, both at the request of the MEB.

KCF has been part of the RIVM since 1996. It is a relatively large group which, on a yearly basis, performs as much work as BTG and FTB together. The KCF originated from the former RIGO (National Institute for Medicine Research), which had been established in 1963, together with the MEB. The RIGO was itself a continuation of the National Institute for Pharmaceutical Therapeutic Research (RIPTO) which had been founded in 1920. Like the preclinical reports, the pharmaceutical evaluation reports were written at that time by a member of the board, until the separation of responsibilities: at a certain point it was considered inappropriate for board members to write reports themselves, as it could be difficult to critically consider a report written by oneself.

In those early days of the MEB, there was already cooperation between the RIV(M) and the RIGO when chemical-pharmaceutical evaluations were involved. This was the result of the original text of the Dutch Medicine Law, which stated that the RIV needed to be consulted on the evaluation of biological aspects. As mentioned earlier, some products of biological origin were considered medicinal products and therefore were evaluated by the RIGO. These were hormones, as porcine insulin for diabetes, and oxytocin. The laboratory research was done by the RIV.

The RIGO had a function in the admission of medicinal products as well as a role in the control of medicinal products after an MA was granted. The RIGO had offices in various locations in Leiden until, in 1996, it merged with the RIVM and its name was changed to the Laboratory for Research of Medicinal Products. It then moved to the RIVM offices in Bilthoven. In 2003, the final name change took place. The current KCF has around 20 evaluators, most of them pharmacists.

The focus of the KCF is on the quality of chemically produced medicinal products. In the Netherlands, as in most other countries, the quality is monitored by the government through a system of licensing and control. The KCF plays an important role, not just in the Netherlands, but increasingly in Europe. KCF employees evaluate applications for MAs and are involved in quality control after the application is granted through laboratory research. At a European level, the KCF plays a role in the maintenance and expansion of the European Pharmacopoeia and the coordination between the national controlling authorities.

Conclusion

Collaboration between the MEB and the RIVM has existed for years. It is dynamic and changes with time. The RIVM not only provides the MEB with evaluators but also with representatives of the MEB on numerous study groups outside the Netherlands, particularly at the EMA. There has always been a lot of influence from other countries and regions, and this will not change. What will also remain unchanged is the great enthusiasm that the RIVM evaluators show, when performing their tasks on behalf of the MEB.

References

[1] *Gezondheidsraad www.gr.nl*
[2] *Directive 89/342 EEC (extending the scope of 65/65/EEC and 75/319/EEC and laying down additional provisions for immunological medicinal products consisting of vaccines, toxins or serums and allergens) and Directive 89/381/EEC (extending the scope of the 65/65/EEC and 75/319/EEC and laying down special provisions for medicinal products derived from human blood or human plasma).*

2025 – will the MEB still be here?

by Frits Lekkerkerker

When passing on the presidency of the MEB to the next incumbent, it is hard to resist philosophising about developments in the registration of medicinal products in the future. There will be significant changes, as there have been in the past 16 years during my presidency. These changes will primarily be at the European level, but will certainly have consequences for the MEB. Changes will happen through national influence too. Core issues are: more decisions at the European level; greater care for safe administration of medicinal products; greater openness and transparency; greater influence of patient organisations and a greater responsibility for society as a whole. At a national level, proper use and optimal use of medicines will require more attention by the MEB. Cost-saving efforts on ensuring that pharmaceutical therapy is as safe as possible require vigilance, so that quality is not jeopardised.

The division between real medicinal products and products with health claims will become blurred, just like the division between indications for medicinal products and health benefits of nutrients. Will the MEB function the same way 15 years from now?

From a historic point of view

In the past 16 years plus, a lot has happened. From a solely national responsibility, the registration of medicines has become a collective responsibility of the EU member states. In 1990, there was a European scientific committee, but the decisions, or rather the recommendations, had to be implemented nationally, and that sometimes happened with national adaptations. This committee was also limited to the evaluation of biotechnological medicinal products. There was a cautious start to mutual recognition of national registrations.

This changed drastically in 1995 with the emergence of the EMA. When this agency came into force (originally as the EMEA), the task of the scientific committee changed. This committee (the CPMP, now CHMP) issued scientific recommendations which were adopted by the European Commission and converted into European decisions virtually unchanged. This meant that admission of new medicinal products happened at the European level, and national authorities could not change that. The European Commission, at its end, has done everything it can to eliminate trade barriers within the EU, in accordance with the goal of the EU. The necessary extensive legislation – Directives and Regulations – have been amended and renewed during the past 16 years. The Netherlands, with their rich history in critical evaluation of medicinal products, was able to greatly influence this European legislation, as their delegates were very active. In this way, the Dutch way of critical scientific evaluation could be continued within Europe.

Registration activities are not limited to the admission of medicinal products to the market. With registration, the official product information is determined, via its SmPC. This SmPC is continuously amended according to new developments or new information about the safe use of the medication. The SmPC is the source of information for physicians and pharmacists about why, how and when to use this medicinal product. The insert meant for patients, the PIL, is based on the SmPC and is determined in the same way. New information on safe use requires amendment of both of these documents. This working method will not change in the coming years. What will change is the way in which the recommendations of the CHMP are created. European expert groups, national experts, and patient representatives will be more involved. The complexity of the decision-making will increase. In recent years, transparency and openness have received a lot of attention, because of the increased complexity of the decisions, and these will therefore need to be increased even more. This will not just be a task for the EMA, but the national registration authorities, which are closer to the various special interest groups, will also have a growing role in the explanation of European legislation.

European procedures

At this point in time medicinal products can be registered through two different European procedures, the CP and the DCP. The CP, in which the EMA has a leading role, was until recently only used for new medicinal products. The DCP, which for each individual product is led by one of the member states, is primarily intended for older medicinal products and generics; this procedure is seldom used for new compounds. As has previously been noted, all of these procedures are supported by a number of European scientific committees. Other than the CHMP, there is the PDCO for paediatric medicines, the COMP for the designation of orphan products and the CAT for gene therapies, to name but a few. The DCP has a coordination group too – the CMD(h). What will change in the years to come, and what can be expected?

The Centralised Procedure (CP)

Experiences in the past several years have taught a few member states to do most of their scientific preparation within the centralised procedure. Out of a total of 27 member states, only about seven states are really active, of which the Netherlands is one. The work is done by two rapporteurs, members of the CHMP, who are nominated for each application or procedure. The preparation consists of the evaluation of the submitted dossier, which results in an evaluation report. After this, decisions are made by the scientific committees. The same member states are also active in the final decision process; luckily, some other members of the CHMP get involved in this process too.

We can expect the CP to increase in importance. Soon, generics and OTC medicines will be registered using the CP too. For OTC products, the MEB will still need to decide how the product will be distributed, ie, sold only at pharmacies or also in grocery stores, gas stations and other generally available outlets.

Will the scientific evaluation be done by more member states in the future? This can be viewed in two ways: From the European point of view it is best if as many member states as possible participate, only then will the European decision process be supported by all member states. On the other hand, it is estimated that only around 40-50 new products will need to be evaluated in any given year, resulting in around 90 rapporteur positions. To keep as much expertise as possible involved in the preparation, the national authorities need to have eight to 12 rapporteurs positions. If they have less, they cannot maintain their expertise, as it becomes less attractive to work for these authorities. It is therefore likely that the current situation will remain, which will require that active countries make efforts to maintain their expertise. That is certainly true for the MEB and its employees.

When nominating rapporteurs, initially each member of the CHMP should have an equal amount of rapporteurships. In reality, some of the members have had little interest in this, which has led to the current lopsided situation. As a result of this, the nomination process has changed. Currently, a national authority must prove it has the required expertise to hold the position. In the coming years this will be viewed more critically. This is good for the development of expertise in the national offices, but it also provides a safety-net so that some countries do not have a monopoly on the assessment of certain products. This could otherwise mean that, for example, anticancer medicines could only be evaluated in two or three countries, which would be an unacceptably one-sided approach.

These developments lead to the expectation that, also in the future, much of the preparation will still be done by a few countries. To reach a pan-European final decision, the level of expertise of the less active member countries needs to be high too. Those members will need to have a clearly defined scientific background, more so than is currently required. They also need to be supported by national experts or a registration authority.

Another possibility is that the London office, the EMA, will do the scientific preparations. In this case, scientific evaluators from the other EU member states need to be recruited. It is not clear if this would benefit the scientific judgment. The drawback here is that the full-time rapporteurs in London would lose touch with daily practice, and the involvement of the individual member states would decrease. A risk also exists that the national authorities would lose expertise and these offices would only have administrative functions. This would not be a good situation, as it could decrease national support. Moreover, the national authorities do need their expertise to maintain their level of pharmacovigilance and their function of promoting safe use of medicines. It is therefore unlikely that this form of centralisation will happen in the next 15 years.

The Decentralised Procedure (DCP)

The DCP will remain important in the coming years. The same countries that are active at centralised level are also active at the decentralised level. This DCP level often concerns older medicinal products and generics, and here especially the quality requirements should be high. This is not easy to maintain with a globalised manufacturing process. Many generic medicinal products are researched and/or produced in developing countries. To guarantee their safety more inspections are needed, and Europe currently lacks the capacity for this. It requires a closer collaboration with other member states, and also with the US FDA. The latter has not been arranged so far, but this needs to been done in the short term.

Safe administration

Safety, and in particular the safe use of medicinal products, will have a strong emphasis in the coming years, as well as greater attention by the press and the politicians. Currently this is a national responsibility in which the EMA only has a coordinating function, which works well because pharmacotherapy is primarily at national level. The Dutch do take their medications differently than people in Southern Europe, but if there is a concern about the safety of a medicine, the measures to deal with should be the same everywhere. This requires European coordination, which can be improved at this point. The European Commission is therefore working on new legislation, and there are plans for a separate scientific committee for pharmacovigilance. Such a committee with its own responsibilities could ease the European decision-making process, although there is a risk that the various committees might contradict each other. This would be true for the CHMP, which currently has a working party that deals with pharmacovigilance, albeit this working party does not have any decision-making authority. Experiences with the coordination of the recommendations have not always been positive, and a separate committee could be useful if there is enough expertise in the committee, as well as expertise from prescribers and consumers. Current experiences with representatives of patient groups in the safety evaluation are positive. The success of the committee will also depend on good communication in which, again, prescribers and consumers need to be involved. The US FDA has great respect from the press and the public, as well as in the Netherlands. The FDA's responsibilities are different from those of the MEB. The MEB operates at a greater distance from the industry. In addition, the use of medicinal products in the US is vastly different from that in Europe, and certainly in the Netherlands. In Europe, no direct-to-consumer advertising is allowed for medicines that are available only on prescription. I think, therefore, that comparisons with the FDA are incorrect, and that it is not right that the FDA should be so highly regarded by the press. Europe and the Netherlands react to safety issues just as adequately as the US, and these actions deserve more attention from the press than is currently given. It would be good to have a more proactive, and less retroactive, approach in Europe, as the media love to send worrying signals out to the public, without thinking of the consequences. It should be clear that not all signals sent by the media are based on complete and reliable analyses of a problem.

Patient representatives

As noted, experiences with patient groups have been very positive, at a European as well as a national level, where working groups consisting of patient representatives and authorities are active. Patient representatives have learned to contribute positively and proactively to recommendations. Their have high-level expertise, much more so than was originally assumed, when such cooperation began. This development will continue with increasing speed. The European COMP and the PDCO already have lay-members. The Dutch MEB, contrary to its British counterpart, does not have patient representation. I do expect discussions about this to begin soon. The hurdle to be surmounted is the confidentiality of the dossiers, but there are already clear agreements on this at an EU level with patient organisations to guarantee confidentiality, and this should be possible in the Netherlands too.

There is, of course, the possibility that the pharmaceutical industries of various countries might have an influence on patient groups, but this is also true with prescribers and even with scientists. The current agreements, of full transparency of financial resources and other requirements for patient representation, should and will be able to avoid this.

Transparency

The press often voices distrust of pharmaceutical companies as well as registration authorities. It talks about the way the evaluations are conducted, and of the influence of the industry on the authorities. The media points to the conflicts of interest of MEB employees and its experts. By itself, this concern is justified. The industry and the registration authorities both like to make use of the best scientists. Conflicts of interest can only be avoided by even greater transparency and the publication of decisions. This will be the great challenge for the MEB and its secretariat. Its communications department dedicates a lot of time to this, but it only has a limited staff. The solution is not just in increasing the number of employees for that department – all employees have to contribute. Creating good scientific reports is different from the communications about them. The latter requires training.

In the past there has been a lot of criticism about the MEB's lack of openness, but this has changed greatly in recent years. The MEB has worked hard to address these criticisms, including creating the new website mentioned in previous chapters, which holds not only an abridged version of the minutes of MEB meetings but also the agendas of these meetings, which are published on the website shortly before the meetings, as well as summaries of the topics discussed.

The industry sometimes objects to such increased transparency and is concerned that this will affect its competitiveness. Pharmaceutical companies, too, will have to learn that public suspicion will only decrease if there is greater transparency. An industry whose job is to search for new ways of treating illnesses should not be mistrusted. The call to leave the development of medicinal products to governments is Utopian, however, particularly given the tremendous financial risks that are involved. Governments will have to facilitate the development of medicinal products, which in fact they already do. There is a need for medicinal products for a great number of diseases that as yet are untreatable, the so-called priority medicines, the development of which need to be stimulated in particular. Consultations with patient advocacy groups and healthcare professionals are important to determine which medicines deserve such priority. There remains a lot to be done in this field.

The goals of greater transparency and more openness are not just aimed at showing the pharmacotherapeutic possibilities, but also at highlighting the risks. This is particularly important for new medicinal products. One of the ways to create a greater openness about risks is the publication of PSURs. The industry is already required to submit the data for these periodic safety reports to the registration authorities for their creation of evaluation reports. And while it is not easy to compile a report that the public, the press and other professionals find easy to understand, they can learn to interpret such reports correctly. This kind of openness is essential to gain an increase in trust in available medicinal products. Publication of PSURs should be a high priority.

The MEB and its support staff

What will change for the MEB and the staff that supports it, the Secretariat, by 2025? The MEB with its 17 members will have a different face. Originally it was a very critical-scientific board consisting of representatives of all disciplines who were involved with the use and development of medicinal products. The MEB took decisions behind closed doors. Slowly they began paying more attention to the social aspects of medicines, and to borderline products such as herbs and homeopathic products – medicines that do have a place in Dutch society today. The MEB's task in this is to ensure these products, too, are safe and can be used in a safe manner. This includes good education. If the MEB wants a reason for its existence it has to be orientated to society. This can also mean that representatives of patient organisations have a seat on the MEB. The MEB is supported by a large number of staff members, the Secretariat. They need special attention. A separate group of employees are the clinical evaluators, and employees of the department of pharmacovigilance. Current policy is aimed at giving these people part-time evaluation tasks and part-time clinical or research tasks. That policy needs to be strengthened. Already some of these individuals have a function at a clinical or oncology centre, or they are employed at a university department for pharmacoepidemiology. This approach assures that the MEB uses experienced employees, who remain in touch with clinical work and research. A close-knit team, the evaluators together with the employees of the Secretariat produce high quality work. However, the MEB needs to supervise the Secretariat, which requires adequate attention.

Contacts in the field are initiated through the members of the MEB. An initiative has begun to create more national expert groups. This development needs to be reinforced. Currently there is a sounding board for paediatricians, and consultations with paediatric psychiatrists have been highly successful. It is important that these experts are also going to be active within Europe on behalf of the CHMP and other scientific committees. The members of the MEB are the most appropriate members for these groups, and good coordination among the other experts, the MEB, and the Secretariat, is essential. – a challenge for the coming years.

Conclusion

The MEB will still be important in 2025, but it will operate differently. Attention to the national market for medicinal products is an important issue. That means attention to pharmacovigilance, but also to education and information. The presence of the MEB in society will increase. Proper coordination with insurance companies on pharmacotherapy is one aspect of this.

It is expected that more registration issues will be dealt with at a European level. Although the Netherlands is not the largest country in the EU – of all 27 members states, seven countries are larger – it will need to keep its grip on European developments, even though it will have less direct influence. The Netherlands has always been strict in its critical evaluations of medicinal products, and so the Dutch voice needs to be heard in Europe in the years to come. That strict stance needs to remain anchored in Europe, and the Netherlands' representatives can contribute to this. Action is needed to ensure the continuation of a strong, albeit indirect, influence. Dutch university institutions have great expertise in the field of clinical pharmacology, on many aspects of clinical medicine and on pharmacoepidemiology, which needs to be applied. Scientific institutions benefit from this, too, and realise this. To leave this application of expertise to the larger countries is not an option.

About the authors

Stan van Belkum has worked in the registration of medicinal products arena for 15 years, initially as quality expert at the RIVM, and later in different positions at the MEB. Over the course of several years he has gained experience in the field of process optimisation and the creation of standard procedures for the exchange of data between the pharmaceutical industry and government. In this last function, he has been internationally active for more than ten years. He has been Topic Leader for the electronic dossier at the ICH, a harmonisation project between the US, the EU and Japan. In the past few years he has focused on establishing the MEB workflow and document management system.

Henk van den Berg is currently working as a paediatric haematologist/oncologist at the Emma Children's Hospital AMC in Amsterdam. As of July 2007, he is Alternate Member of the EMA's Paediatric Committee, the PDCO. He trained in paediatrics at the Academic Hospital of the University of Amsterdam (currently the Academic Medical Centre). He was registered as a paediatrician in 1984. During his employment in the paediatric department of the Leiden University Hospital, on the paediatric ward for bone marrow transplantation, he completed his PhD at the Leiden State University in 1991. His thesis was titled: 'Reconstitution of Hematopoieses after Allogeneic Bone Marrow Transplantation in Children.' He was one of the editors of the paediatric formulary of the Academic Medical Centre.

Liesbeth Breeveld is head of the Department of Information and Communication at the MEB, and is responsible for the internal and external communications policy. This includes roles as spokesperson, coordination of external contacts, communications advice and the various means of communication such as the website and the intranet. Prior to her position at the MEB, she was Corporate Communications Manager at Leerdammer Company and senior communications adviser at Paul Kok Consultants, with principal roles in the nutrition branch, healthcare and the pharmaceutical industry. Liesbeth graduated from the Amsterdam University where she studied European Studies and from the course entitled 'Corporate communications in business administrative aspects' at the Erasmus University, Rotterdam.

Emiel van Galen is responsible for the evaluation of homeopathic, anthroposophic and herbal medicinal products at the MEB. He is head of the Department of Botanicals and Novel Foods at the agency of the MEB. In the past decade he participated in various working groups at European level, focused on the evaluation of these medicinal products in the EU. As of 2004 he represents the Netherlands on the Herbal Medicinal Products Committee at the European Medicines Agency in London, UK. Since 2007 he has been chair of the Homeopathic Medicinal Products Working Group (HMPWG), of the Heads of Medicines Agencies, a group for harmonisation of assessment criteria and for exchange of regulatory experiences concerning homeopathics between member states.

Pim van der Giesen studied pharmacy at the State University of Utrecht and obtained his PhD at the same university. He has worked at the MEB since 1988 in various positions. He was a member of the EU Committee of Human Medicinal Products (CHMP) on behalf of the Netherlands between 1995 and 2002 at the EMA (formerly the EMEA) in London, UK. Until 2009 he was a member of the Pharmacovigilance Working Party (PhVWP) at the EMA on behalf of the MEB.

Kees van Grootheest is Director of the Netherlands Pharmacovigilance Centre Lareb and Professor of Pharmacovigilance at the State University in Groningen. He studied medicine at the Free University, Amsterdam. He has previously worked as general physician in the Netherlands and in developing countries.

Josée Hansen is chief inspector at the Netherlands Healthcare Inspectorate (IGZ). She is responsible for the control of medicinal products, medical devices, blood, tissue and organs. From May 2007 until early 2010 she was project leader at the WHO in Geneva of the Priority Medical Devices project. From 2002 until 2005 she was acting Inspector General for Health Care. During this period she chaired the task force for patient safety of the Dutch Health Care inspectorate. From 1991 until 1999 she was senior inspector, and coordinated the hospital inspections of medical devices among other assignments. She studied pharmacy at the State University in Utrecht. After graduation she worked as a community pharmacist including hospital pharmacy.

Yechiel (Chiel) Hekster has been Professor, Clinical Pharmacy, at the Radboud University Nijmegen Medical Centre since 1998. He is also responsible for the education of hospital pharmacists in his department. In addition, he is a member of the MEB and head of the scientific advice Committee (WAR) of the Lareb. He is editor of a number of scientific periodicals. He studied pharmacy in Leiden and obtained his PhD in Nijmegen. He has been active in the European Society of Clinical Pharmacy (ESCP), where he chaired the research and Education Committee and was President of the society.

Arno Hoes is Professor, Clinical Epidemiology and General Medicine, at the Utrecht Medical Centre, where he is also manager of research. He studied medicine at the Catholic University in Nijmegen. He obtained his PhD at the Erasmus University in Rotterdam, and continued his specialty at the London School of Hygiene and Tropical Medicine. In 1991, he became Assistant Professor in Clinical Epidemiology at the Erasmus Medical Centre. His education experience includes classes in the field of research design, clinical epidemiology, diagnostic research, evidence-based medicine and coronary diseases. He has been employed by the MEB since 1998.

Truus Janse-de Hoog has been head of the Coordination Group for Mutual Recognition and Decentralised Procedures – human (CMD(h)) since 2005. She is a staff member of the Cluster Group, EU. After studying chemistry and pharmacy, she worked first as a pharmacist and later as a hospital pharmacist. She joined the MEB in October 1989, and in 1991 she was nominated adjunct secretary. In 1995, she became the Dutch representative at the Mutual Recognition Facilitation Group (MRFG), the European consultation group for mutual recognition procedures.

Aginus Kalis has been Secretary of the MEB since 2004 and Executive Director of the Agency. He also represents the Netherlands as Member of the Management Board of the EMA in London and is Chairman of the Management Group of Heads of Medicines Agencies. He is a member of the Advisory Council for The Organisation for Professionals in Regulatory Affairs (TOPRA). After completing his medical studies at the Erasmus University in Rotterdam, he was first a physician and later a transplant coordinator. In 1990, he became Medical Director of Duphar, the Netherlands (later Solvay Pharma, the Netherlands). In 1997, he joined the Care Management department at Silver Cross/Achmea. In 1999, he transferred to the public sector and became Director, Healthcare Management, at the Dutch Department of Health.

Bert Klijn is Advisor, External Communications, at the MEB. At a young age he became a freelance journalist/correspondent at various daily and weekly publications. Following an interim period as a cultural professional, he rejoined the ranks of freelance/scientific journalists. In 1998, he joined the MEB as an editor. In 2005, he transferred to the Department of Information and Communication at the MEB to organise internal communications.

Jan Willem van der Laan has been employed at the National Institute for Public Health and the Environment (RIVM) since 1980. He worked initially as a pharmacologist/evaluator of CNS products. As of 1990, he has been coordinator of the pharmacological/toxicological evaluations for the MEB, and as such he is also a member of the Safety Working Party. As of 1992 he has taken part in the ICH process on carcinogenics as a member of the Expert / Working Group and later on the Immune-toxicity rapporteur. In September/October 1995 he worked at the FDA as a temporary employee. He obtained his PhD on a bio-chemical/behaviour pharmacological topic at the Pharmacology Group of the Medical Department of the Erasmus University of Rotterdam.

Frits Lekkerkerker was Director of the MEB from 1991 until 2007. He was a member of the CHMP Working Parties on biosimilars and contact with patient groups. As Director he had a special interest in the responsibility of the MEB towards society. He is a physician of internal medicine, and did his PhD research on calcium metabolism. He worked in the endocrinology department of hospitals in Groningen and Enschede, as supervisor of the merger of the departments of internal medicine of both hospitals. For many years he was head of the Commission Incidents Patient Care (MIP). He first became a member of the MEB in 1974, and was closely involved with its reorganisation in 1986. In 1988, he became vice president and member of the Benelux Committee for Medicinal Products.

Bert Leufkens has been Director of the MEB since 2007. He studied pharmacy at the State University of Utrecht, and later worked for some time at universities in Leiden and Minneapolis (US). In 1987, he contributed to the development of the department of pharmacoepidemiology at the Utrecht Institute for Pharmaceutical Sciences (UIPS). In 1997, he became Professor at this Institute. From 2006–2007 he was head of the Department of Pharmaceutical Sciences. He has a broad interest in pharmaceutical innovation, registration, policy-making, and pharmacovigilance. He is (co)-author of more than 250 scientific publications.

Raymond Meijer is a staff advisor at the MEB and functions as Secretary at the MEB meetings. He has focused more and more on the judiciary over the years, because of the possibilities in the appeal procedures. He studied physics and chemistry at the University of Amsterdam. He obtained his PhD researching the electric, magnetic and thermal properties of the inter-metallic compound indium-bismuth. He taught mathematics for one year before starting his studies in pharmacy at the University of Amsterdam. After graduation he was employed at the secretariat of the MEB, originally as part of the inspection process.

Melita van der Mersch is an attorney at the law firm Pels Rijcken & Droogleever Fortuijn. She specialises in pharmaceutical law, focusing on advice and conflicts about registrations of medicinal products and the reimbursement thereof. She is a board member of the Society for Pharmacy and Law, and editor of the periodicals Health Care Jurisprudence and Pharma Law. In 2006, she wrote part of the preliminary report of the Society for Health Care Law with co-author Caren Velink.

Hans Ovelgönne is currently the Dutch member of the Committee for Advanced Therapies at the EMA. He also represents the MEB in the Gene Therapy Working Party and the Scientific Advice Working Party at the EMA. Until recently, he was head of the department for Quality of Biologic Medicines (KBG) of the RIVM. He obtained his PhD from the department of molecular cell biology at Utrecht University. He held research positions at the veterinary and biology departments of Utrecht University and at the departments of avian virology and mammal virology at the ID-DLO in Lelystad.

Jan M van Ree has been Professor, Psychopharmacology, since 1987, and since 2001 has also held the position of Director of the Rudolf Magnus Institute for Neurosciences of the University Hospital of the State University, Utrecht, which researches pharmacology, neurosurgery, neurology, neurosciences and psychiatry. He started in 1969 at the Rudolf Magnus Institute for Pharmacology and specialised in this field. In 1975 he obtained his PhD conducting research on the effect of psychoactive compounds in rats. He was also involved in organising congresses in the field of (psycho)pharmacology in the Netherlands and in Europe, he was member of the MEB, founder of the Hersenstichting Nederland and the Nederlands Hersendecennium (both institutes focus on public awareness of brain function). He was also head of the central commission of treatment of heroin addicts and chief editor of the scientific publication, European Neuropsychopharmacology.

Jan Schellens is Internal Medicine Physician-Oncologist-Clinical Pharmacologist at the Netherlands Cancer Institute – Antoni van Leeuwenhoek Hospital (NKI–AVL) in Amsterdam, and Professor, Medicinal Toxicology, of beta faculty department of pharmaceutical sciences of the State University of Utrecht. He is head of the department of clinical pharmacology of the NKI-AVL. He is an educator for the focus field Clinical Pharmacology for internal medicine physicians, which is hosted by the Dutch Society for Internal Medicine Physicians. He is president of the Dutch Society for Clinical Pharmacology & Bio-pharmacy. He is a member of the MEB and head of the Commission for Pharmaceutical Help of the College of Health Insurances (CVZ).

Fred Schobben is Professor, Clinical Pharmacotherapy, at the department of pharmaceutical sciences of the State University in Utrecht. He is also a hospital pharmacist and clinical pharmacologist at the University Hospital in Utrecht, and coordinator of the pharmacology/pharmacotherapy education of the masters degree for medicine. He has been a member of the MEB since 1988, and was deputy head of the MEB between 1995 and 2006. He has a special interest in the broad field of pharmacotherapy, the medical, ethical, and scientific evaluation of medicinal products.

Diederick Slijkerman has been head of Policy and Legal Affairs at the MEB since late 2009. He took the initiative for this book and is the editor. After completing his studies in Law and History at the State University in Leiden, he worked for the state government and various industries. He has published on multiple topics in periodicals and daily newspapers and is currently working on his PhD research. He represents the MEB at the EMACOLEX, a consultancy of legal and policy-making experts from the European member states, the EMA, and the European Commission. In 2005 he became part-time staff advisor at the MEB. In 2006 he was nominated adjunct secretary of the MEB. He was also MEB project leader for the creation of a new system for homecare products.

Sabine Straus has been head of the department of pharmacovigilance at the MEB since late 2005. She started her career at the MEB in 1997 as a senior evaluator in pharmacovigilance. She studied medicine at the State University in Utrecht and graduated in 1985. She has previously worked for various pharmaceutical companies; her last position was at Searle Monsanto where she was Medical Director. In 2004 she obtained a Master of Science degree in Clinical Epidemiology at the Erasmus University in Rotterdam. She obtained her PhD in 2005 in Rotterdam. Her thesis was entitled: 'Medicines, QTC Extension and Acute Heart Failure'.

Jan Taminiau is a paediatrician and paediatric gastroenterologist. In 1991 he was involved in the creation of the Medicine Reimbursement System for paediatric medicines and he has since been a member of the Commission Pharmaceutical Help of the Public Health Insurance (later, the CVZ). He has been a member of the MEB since 2005, and as of 2007 he represents the MEB at the Paediatric Committee of the EMA in London. He is involved in medicines research in children at the children's hospital of the University Hospital of the Amsterdam University. He is involved in pharmacokinetic studies and clinical studies (EU/US) in the field of paediatric gastroenterology, hepatology, and nutrition.

Frank Verheijen is head of the Department of Veterinary Medicine at the MEB. He studied biology at the Agricultural University in Wageningen, specialising in Animal Production and Health Science. After graduating he worked for more than ten years as scientific project leader at the Department of Pharmacological R&D of Intervet International on the development of veterinary medicines. He was head of the department of swine and poultry-keeping of the Innovation and Practice Centre (IPC) in Barneveld. Later he became marketing manager/senior researcher at the business unit Agrisystems and Environment of Wageningen-UR.

Bettie Voordouw is chief evaluator of the clinical department of the MEB. She is the Dutch representative at the Committee for Orphan Medicinal Products (COMP) at the EMA in London, and observer at the focus group for Orphan Drugs (WGN). She is a member of various other organisations such as the World Health Organisation (WHO) and the European Centre for Disease Preventions and Control (ECDC). Her background is in medicine and she holds a masters degree in public health. Her thesis was about research of efficacy of the annual influenza vaccination campaign in people 65 years and older.

Waldo Weijers is a staff advisor at the MEB and acts as Secretary at meetings of the Agency. He is also coordinator of the consultation procedures for medical devices with a pharmaceutical compound. These procedures are being done by the MEB and the notified bodies. He graduated with a degree in pharmacy at the State University in Utrecht in 1992. He worked as a pharmacist in Rotterdam and taught at the Utrecht University before joining the MEB. He worked initially as a chemical-pharmaceutical evaluator, and later as a registration coordinator.

Barbara van Zwieten-Boot has been a member of the CHMP on behalf of the Netherlands since 2001. She has experience at universities as well as in the pharmaceutical industry and the MEB. She obtained her PhD at the State University of Utrecht, where she also did an additional year of research. She was employed at Rhone-Poulenc for seven years. In this position she gained experience in starting and supervising clinical research and the registration of medicinal products. Following this she transferred to government agencies. She worked at the MEB as clinical evaluator of primarily CNS products. As a member, and later as head of the Efficacy Working Party, and as clinical content coordinator for the EU at ICH, she made a case for the harmonisation of the clinical requirements for registration.

Glossary of abbreviations

ADME: Absorption, distribution, metabolism and elimination [or excretion]

ADR: Adverse drug reaction

AV: Generally available [medications]

BfArM: Germany's Federal Institute for Drugs and Medical Devices (Bundesinstitut fuer Arzneimittel und Medicinal Produkte)

BMT: State Laboratory for Biological Medicines [a department within the RIVM]

BPWP: Blood Products Working Party

BTG: Bio-Technological Medicinal Products [a section within the RIVM]

BWP: Biologics Working Party

CAT: Committee for Advanced Therapies

CBER: Centre for biologics evaluation and research (US)

CBG: The competent authority to assess risk/benefit and for issuing marketing authorisations of medicinal products

CCMO: (Centrale Commissie Mensgebonden Onderzoek): the competent authority for assessing clinical trials

CDER: Centre for drug evaluation and research (US)

CHMP: Committee for Human Medicinal Products

CMD: Coordination Group for Mutual Recognition Procedures and Decentralised Procedures

CMD(h): Coordination Group for MRP and Decentralised Procedures – Human

CMD(v): Coordination Group for MRP and Decentralised Procedures – Veterinary

CMS: Concerned member state

COMP: Committee for Orphan Medicinal Products

CP: Centralised procedure

CPMP: Committee for Proprietary Medicinal Products

CPWP: Cell-based Products Working Party

CTD: Common Technical Document

CVMP: Committee for Veterinary Medicinal Products

DATHUG: Databank of Human Medicines

DCP: Decentralised procedure

DHPC: Direct Healthcare Professional Communication (formerly 'Dear Doctor Letter')

EEA: European Economic Area

EMA: European Medicines Agency

EWG: Expert Working Group

EWP: Efficacy Working Party

FTB: Pharmacological-Toxicological Evaluations [a section within the RIVM]

FTE: Full-time equivalent

GDP: Good Distribution Practice

GMP: Good Manufacturing Practice

GMT: Directorate of Medicines and Medical Technology of the Dutch Ministry for Public Health, Welfare and Sport

GPP: Good Paediatric Practice

GRB: Global Regulatory Board

GTWP: Gene Therapy Working Party

HMA: Heads of Medicines Agencies

HMPC: Herbal Medicinal Products Committee

ICH: International Conference of Harmonisation

ICSR: Individual Case Safety Report

ICT: Information and Communication Technology

IGZ: The Netherlands Healthcare Inspectorate

KCF: Centre for Quality of Chemical-Pharmaceutical Products [a department within the RIVM]

KEMA: The notified body for the Netherlands

KNMG: The Royal Dutch Medicine Organisation

KNMP: The Royal Dutch Association for the Advancement of Pharmacy

KZ: Quality in Healthcare Act /Quality of Healthcare Institutions Act

LAGRA-9: The 9th Local Affiliate of the Global Regulatory Authority

Lareb: Netherlands Pharmacovigilance Centre

LIM: Lareb Intensive Monitoring [a new form of pharmacovigilance]

MA: Marketing authorisation

MAH: Marketing authorisation holder

MCRN: Dutch Medicines Research Network

MEB: Agency of the Dutch Medicines Evaluation Board

MRFG: Mutual Recognition Procedure Facilitation Group

MRP: Mutual Recognition Procedure

MUMS: Minor use in minor species

NKFK: Dutch Centre of Pharmacotherapy in Children

NOAEL: No observable adverse effect level

NOEL: No observable effect level

NSAIDs: Nonsteroidal anti-inflammatory drugs

OTC: Over-the-counter [non-prescription medication]

PCWP: Patients' and Consumers' Working Party

PDCO: Paediatrics Committee

PEI: Paul-Ehrlich-Institut, a division of Germany's Federal Ministry of Health

PgWP: Pharmacogenics Working Party

Ph Eur: European Pharmacopoeia

PhVWP: Pharmacovigilance Working Party

PIL: Patient Information Leaflet

PIP: Paediatric investigation plan

PMS: Post-marketing surveillance

PUMA: Paediatric-use marketing authorisation

PSUR: Periodic safety update report

QWP: Quality Working Party

RCL: State Control Laboratories [a department within the RIVM]

RMP: Risk management plan

RMS: Reference member state

RIGO: National Institute for Medicine Research

RIVM: Dutch National Institute for Public Health and the Environment

SAG: Scientific Advisory Group

SAWP: Scientific Advice Working Party

SC: Steering Committee

SmPC: Summary of Product Characteristics [aka SPC]

STD: Sexually Transmitted Disease

SWP: Safety Working Party

TCM: Traditional Chinese medicine

TSE: Transmittable spongiform encephalopathy

UA: Pharmacy Only [medications]

UAD: Pharmacy and Drugstore [medications]

VWP: Vaccine Working Party

VWS: Health and Public Welfare and Sport

WHO: World Health Organisation

Index of figures and tables

About TOPRA

The past three decades have seen the importance of healthcare regulatory affairs rise to an all-time high. Regulatory professionals are pivotal to the successful development and bringing to market of innovative medicines and healthcare products to patients. They are also key in developing and implementing surveillance systems to monitor the safety of medicines already on the market.

Many regulatory professionals are members of TOPRA. The Organisation for Professionals in Regulatory Affairs is the global association for regulatory professionals and for those who have an interest in the regulation of pharmaceutical and medical technologies in the healthcare sector.

TOPRA members are drawn from more than 40 countries and members worldwide are actively involved in delivering the services needed by busy regulatory specialists. Members work in a range of healthcare settings, from industry, to the regulatory agencies and the consultancy community. All regulatory sectors are represented, including medical technologies, biotech, veterinary medicines, medical devices, borderline products and pharmaceuticals.

TOPRA is a non-profit, non-political organisation, which seeks to advance the status of the regulatory profession through education and provision of information to its members. Members can benefit from structured training programmes, ranging from intensive introductory courses for new entrants to the profession, through to detailed practical courses on topics of interest to those with a few years' experience, to an MSc qualification.

TOPRA's vision is to be the professional organisation providing high quality education, training, information, support services and networking opportunities for those involved in all aspects of healthcare regulatory affairs supporting individuals in their career development and promoting the profession as a whole.

For more information on TOPRA, membership and information about pharmaceutical and medical technology regulation go to www.topra.org or email topra@topra.org